NEONATAL AND PAEDIATRIC RADIOLOGY CASES

Chief Editor

Dr Khalid Khan FRCR
Consultant Paediatric Radiologist
BHR Hospitals NHS Trust
Romford
London

Co-Editor

Dr Sarah Abdulla FRCR
Consultant Radiologist
BHR Hospitals NHS Trust
Romford
London

Grosvenor House
Publishing Limited

This book is published by
Grosvenor House Publishing Ltd
Link House
140 The Broadway, Tolworth, Surrey, KT6 7HT.
www.grosvenorhousepublishing.co.uk

A CIP record for this book
is available from the British Library

ISBN 978-1-78623-308-0

This book is dedicated to my teacher and my mentor

Dr Ian Kenny FRCR

Previously Consultant Paediatric Radiologist at
The Royal Alexandra Hospital for sick children in Brighton.

I would also like to thank my Wife

Farkhanda Khan

Who supported me throughout the creation of this handbook

Paediatric Radiology Cases

Dr Khalid Khan, BSc, MBBS, FFR, RCSI, MSc (Nuclear Med) FRCR

Dr Sarah Abdulla, BA MBBS MA (Cantab) FRCR

Preface

The diseases encountered in Paediatric Radiology differ from adult Radiology and require extensive sub-specialty knowledge. Paediatric Radiology is therefore, practiced primarily in tertiary medical centres where it exists as an expanding sub-specialty. Outside such centres Paediatric imaging is kept to a minimum and patients are frequently referred to tertiary centres for further investigations and management.

However, as long as there are children and neonates being treated in the hospital there will be exposure to Paediatric Radiology and a basic knowledge of most common pathologies is essential. This is especially true given the evolvement of the sophisticated non-invasive imaging techniques and the explosive growth of intervention radiology. More and more radiology is becoming crucial to the management and diagnosis of paediatric patients. With this in mind I have collected, and I am now sharing the most common and interesting cases I have encountered in my district general hospital.

The target audience for this book includes practicing radiologists, radiology registrars and other physicians and staff treating paediatric patients who can use it as a guide for common paediatric and neonatal conditions. This book has been formatted into chapters based on different systems with the most common and most interesting cases we have encountered in our clinical practice. We hope to add more to each system in our second edition, which we aim to publish in the next few years.

This handbook is only a brief and simplified guide and it is by no means a substitute for larger textbooks on neonatal and paediatric radiology.

We aim to donate a certain percentage to save the children fund for each book that is sold.

Care has been taken to confirm the accuracy of information presented and as far as possible to correct any errors that may have occurred inadvertently.

Dr Khalid Khan Chief Editor

Paediatric and neonatal radiology is often considered a vast and bewildering sub-specialty. My hope is that this book proves a useful guide to all those struggling with paediatric imaging as I have learnt a lot researching and composing it.

This project would not have been possible without the collaboration of paediatric physicians and other radiologists and I thank them all for their hard work.

Dr Sarah Abdulla Co Editor

Foreword

Training in radiology, particularly in preparation for exams such as the FRCR, requires exposure to a large number of cases, combined with relevant teaching. The 3-4 years of training undertaken prior to final exams is simply insufficient to build such exposure, and the trainee must augment their clinical experience through other means. Books such as this excellent collection of paediatric cases can help serve this purpose.

One of the great attractions of paediatrics and paediatric radiology is the wide array of pathology encountered; there are very few 'common' disorders in childhood presenting to the radiologist, and rare disease, seen collectively, is paradoxically common. This is reflected in the delightfully varied case mix presented herein, covering the full range of organ systems.

As a trainee I snapped up all case collections such as this one; I am sure if I were preparing again for the Final FRCR, I would add this book to my library.

Dr Alistair D Calder, FRCR
Consultant Radiologist
Great Ormond Street Hospital for Children NHS Foundation Trust

Acknowledgements

It would not have been possible to the seemingly endless project of this book without the help of many of my colleagues whose names appear below.

My Consultant Paediatric colleague Dr Bagtharia who had commitments to many other projects conceived the idea of the book and he could not help me with the book.

It would not have been possible to begin writing this book without the monumental help from my colleague Mr. Valentine Okeke who helped me to start this venture. He helped me to resize the images and make the required adjustments to shift the images and the texts to arrange them in different formats.

Dr Adeel Haq from the Norwich training scheme who was in neuroradiology training at that time contributed significantly to the computing aspects of this book.

Dr Timothy Ariyanayagam was another neuroradiology trainee to our hospital from Norwich who was the first contributor to our book. His effort of writing and computing 20 excellent and interesting neuroradiology cases is greatly appreciated.

Special note of gratitude goes out to Dr Balkrishna Sharma Consultant Paediatrician who contributed and edited the chest section of the neonatal cases with particular emphasis on clinical aspects. His work was indeed very helpful.

I would like to express my appreciation to Dr Ambalika Das Consultant Paediatrician who deserves a special mention and who helped to write several cases on neonatal gastroenterology, which are of exceptional quality.

Dr Gemma Priego needs a mention for help in writing a few excellent cases.

Dr Alaadin Hamad has written a couple of congenital abnormalities.

Special thanks to Mrs. Priya Peiris for the first proof reading of the book.

Dr Trevor Gaunt who spent three months as short paediatric training in Queens Hospital has contributed to the MSK section of the book.

Last but not the least my appreciation is to Dr Sarah Abdulla Consultant radiologist who appeared on the scene when I had collected all the images and the book had to be put together in a suitable format.

Dr Abdullah worked tirelessly on this venture for at least 12 months and she was finally instrumental in completing the entire project into a format of a complete book.

My acknowledgements cannot be complete without mentioning the name Dr Sanjiv Chawda my neuroradiology colleague who was kind enough to give me all the cases of neuroradiology that have been included in the first section of this book

A final word of thanks to the readership who I hope will enjoy this book.

Dr Khalid Khan FRCR Chief Editor

Please send your comments and feedback to my email address khalid247@gmail.com.

Table of Contents

Neuroradiology cases

Case 1

Dr Timothy Ariyanayagam

An 8-month-old infant presents with a cutaneous naevus overlying the lumbosacral spine.

What is the examination and what are your findings?

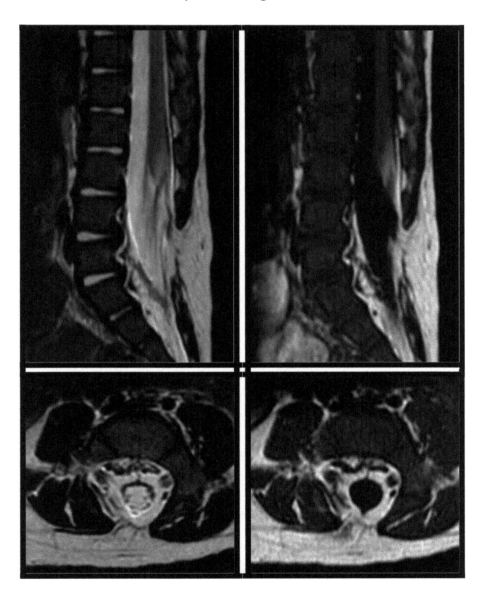

Spinal Dysraphism

Findings: There is evidence of an incomplete vertebral arch posteriorly at L5. There is skin overlying this, in keeping with a closed spinal dysraphism. Of note, there is a terminal lipoma, seen as a discrete area of high T1 and T2 signal on the sagittal images, and low-lying conus, suggestive of a tethered cord.

Discussion: Spinal dysraphism is a term given to a group of dorsal, midline embryological malformations involving mesenchymal, osseous or nervous tissue. This is a heterogeneous group, which includes neural tube defects (e.g. spina bifida).

Spinal dysraphisms may be described as closed or open depending on whether the neural tissue is exposed externally. Spina bifida refers to the bony defect of the vertebral arch, which can allow herniation of various structures.

Closed spinal dysraphisms can include spina bifida occulta, with no other features. This is a relatively common incidental finding, which may or may not be associated with a dimple/hairy tuft/cutaneous abnormality. Other closed dysraphisms include meningocele, dastematomyelia, dorsal dermal sinus, spinal lipoma, or myelocystocoele (a rare dilatation of the central canal which herniates through the dorsal spinal defect).

Open spinal dysraphisms may involve a meningocele, myelocele or myelomeningocele, through a spina bifida aperta

Case 2

Dr Timothy Ariyanayagam

A 10-year-old Afro-Caribbean male presents with severe bone pain that was not relieved by analgesia.

What is the examination and what are your findings?

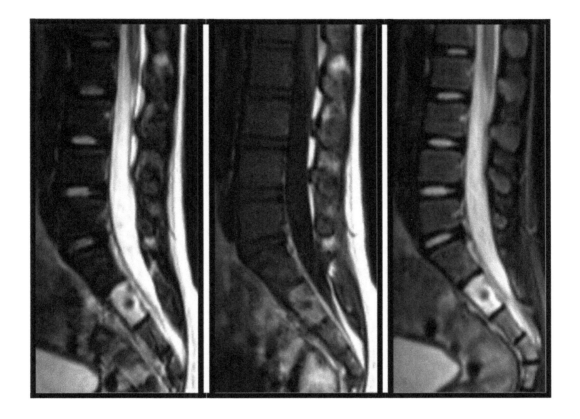

Sickle Cell Crisis – Acute Bone Infarct

Findings: High T2 and STIR signal in the vertebral body of S2 are in keeping with oedema secondary to an acute bone infarct. There is also high T1 signal, which is likely to represent concurrent haemorrhage.

Discussion: Sickle Cell disease is an autosomal recessive chronic haemolytic anaemia, consequent to a single nucleotide polymorphism resulting in the substitution of valine for glutamate at position 6 of the β haemoglobin chain on chromosome 11. This allows the polymerisation of haemoglobin at low oxygen tension, which in turn causes erythrocytes to transform into a rigid sickle shape. This can give rise to vaso-occlusive sickle cell crises as these rigid red blood cells cause stasis of blood and sequestration. One such skeletal manifestation is bone infarction, which typically present as severe bone crises but may be asymptomatic.

In infants and young children between 6 months and 2 years of age these bone crises most often happen in the small tubular bones of the hands and feet causes sickle cell dactylitis or "hand-foot" syndrome. In older children and adults, the long bones are more commonly involved.

Bone infarct and necrosis, along with the hyposplenism that complicates sickle cell anaemia, can lead to osteomyelitis and septic arthritis

Case 3

Dr Timothy Ariyanayagam

A 15-year-old female patient presents with lower back pain.

What are the examinations and what are your findings?

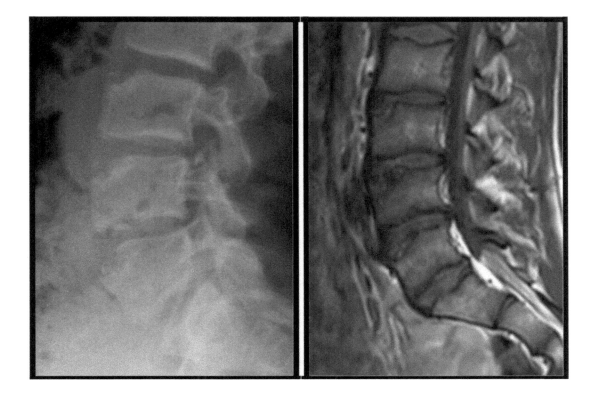

Limbus Vertebra

Findings: The plain radiograph (above left) shows well corticated osseous densities at the anterosuperior corners of L3, L4 and L5. The sagittal T1 image (above right) demonstrates the corresponding lesions with herniation of disc material between the depressed anterior end plate and the apophysis.

Discussion: A limbus vertebra is caused by herniation of the nucleus pulposus of the disc through the apophyseal ring of the vertebra. This results in a well corticated apophysis. This is most commonly seen at the anterosuperior corner.

Anterior limbus vertebrae are said to be asymptomatic.

Case 4

Dr Timothy Ariyanayagam

A 14-year-old male presents with exertional headaches.

What is the diagnosis?

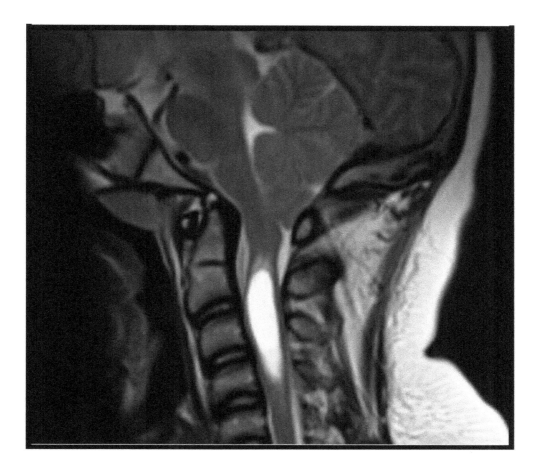

Chiari I Malformation with syrinx

Findings: The T2-weighted sagittal slice shows tonsillar ectopia of 13mm and associated syringomyelia at the level of C2-C4.

Discussion: Chiari I malformations are defined as caudal cerebellar tonsillar ectopia, of greater than 5mm. The precise level of descent is variable depending on age, and children between the ages of 5 – 15 years have greater ectopia than adults or infants, and thus asymptomatic tonsillar herniation of up to 6mm should not be considered pathological in this group. Herniation of less than 5mm can be considered as benign tonsillar ectopia.

There are several possible causes. The most common subgroup of patients has small posterior fossae. Other potential causes include the possible early closure of sutures following ventriculoperitoneal shunt placement, and abnormalities of the foramen magnum such as basilar invagination.

The majority of Chiari I malformations are asymptomatic, and if symptomatic, tend to present in adulthood. The symptoms include occipital headaches on coughing or exertion. 25-35% of patients will have associated syringomyelia, secondary to impeded CSF flow, which may or may not be symptomatic.

Case 5

Dr Timothy Ariyanayagam

An adolescent patient presents with left-sided partial seizures and olfactory hallucinations.

What is the imaging abnormality? Is it related to the patient's symptoms?

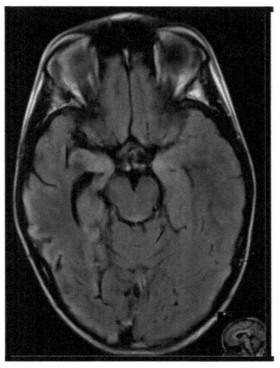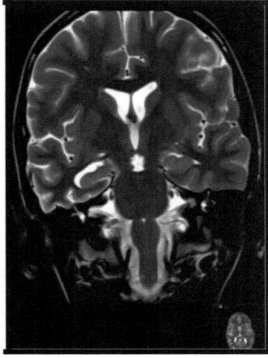

Mesial Temporal Sclerosis

Findings: The coronal T2WI (above right) demonstrates hippocampal volume loss on the right, with the FLAIR images (above left) showing high signal in the hippocampus. The imaging findings are suggestive of mesial temporal sclerosis (MTS).

Discussion: MTS is commonly associated with intractable temporal lobe epilepsy (TLE). This is particularly true of autopsy studies, and imaging findings are seen less frequently. The relationship is also not entirely understood, and it is not known whether MTS is a cause or consequence of TLE.

In this patient, the abnormality is unilateral, and therefore made more obvious by comparing the two sides, however 10% of cases are bilateral. On imaging there is a change in signal and size of the hippocampus which is smaller with a higher T2 / FLAIR signal.

Case 6

Dr Timothy Ariyanayagam

A 13-year-old female presents with bilateral worsening sensorineural hearing loss.

What is the abnormality? Is it related to the patient's symptoms?

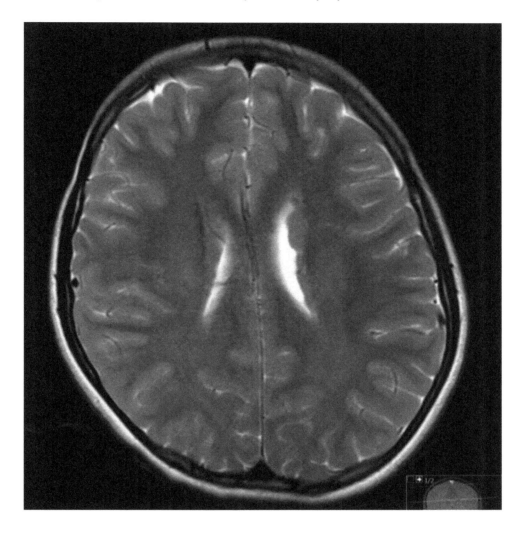

Grey Matter Heterotopia

Findings: There is irregularity of the lateral borders of the ventricles with lesions of similar signal intensity to the grey matter.

Discussion: Grey matter heterotopia is abnormally located collections of nerve cells, secondary to neuronal radial migration arrest. These patients usually present with seizures. There are subtypes based on the location and pattern.

- x Nodular heterotopias
  - o Subependymal
  - o Subcortical
- x Diffuse heterotopias
  - o Band heterotopia
  - o Lissencephaly

Subependymal heterotopias demonstrate cells within the residual germinal zone located *within* the ventricle. These appear as smooth, ovoid masses which are isointense with grey matter on all sequences. There are broadly 2 main groups. Most patients have asymmetrical heterotopia largely confined to the trigones, temporal or occipital horns. These are usually not familial though they may be associated with other anomalies such as Chiari II malformations. A few patients have many heterotopic foci that essentially line the walls of the lateral ventricles. This group may be familial or sporadic.

Our case demonstrates an incidental finding of subependymal heterotopia on the left, in a patient who presented with bilateral sensorineural hearing loss.

Case 7

Dr Timothy Ariyanayagam

A 10-week-old male presents as a floppy infant with a prominent forehead.

What is the diagnosis?

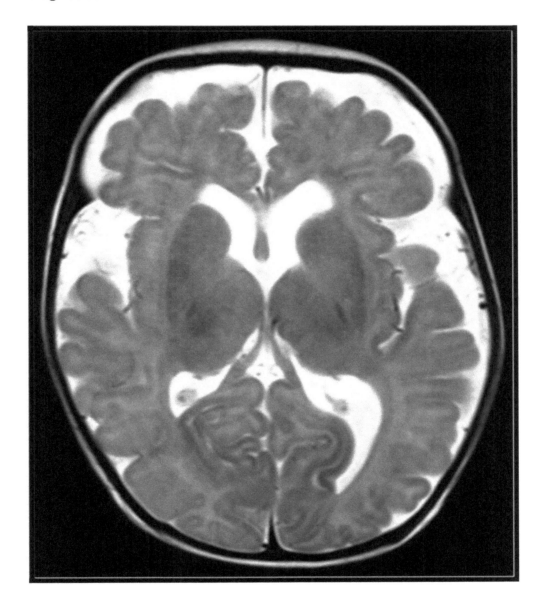

Glutaric Aciduria Type I

Findings: The frontotemporal CSF spaces are enlarged. There is high T2 signal in the basal ganglia and the periventricular white matter.

Discussion: Glutaric Aciduria Type I is an autosomal recessive mitochondrial disorder. There is a deficiency of glutaryl-CoA dehydrogenase, affecting the ability of the mitochondria to metabolise L-lysine, L-hydroxylysine and L-tryptophan. It affects both the white matter and the grey matter, specifically the basal ganglia, most commonly the putamen. Most patients present with an acute encephalopathy by the age of 12 months, often following acute infection or catabolic state, and may demonstrate macrocephaly, hypotonia, progressive dystonia or choreoathetosis, and tetraplegia. After the acute illness, most motor skills will be lost with resultant severe dystonia.

As the disease progresses, there is worsening atrophy, and these patients are susceptible to subdural haemorrhage with minor trauma.

This condition is screened with a neonatal heel prick test performed on infants in the UK.

Case 8

Dr Timothy Ariyanayagam

A 16-year-old male presents with two left sided partial seizures.

What is the imaging abnormality?

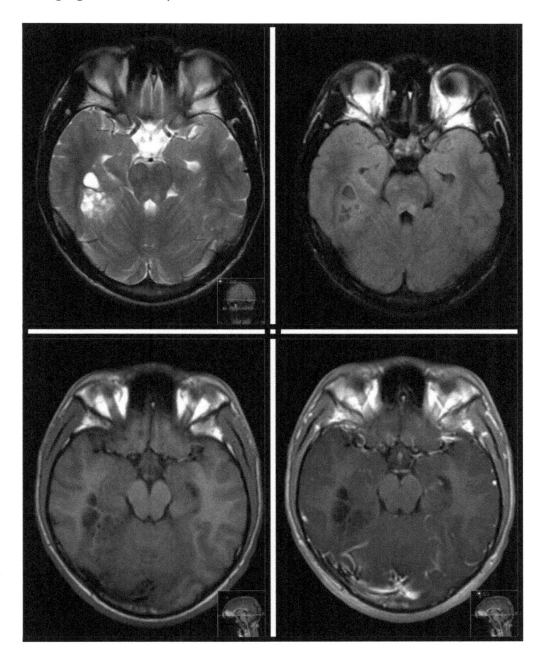

Case 8

Dysembryoplastic Neuroepithelial Tumour (DNET)

Findings: Imaging findings are of high T2 signal "bubbly" lesion, corresponding low T1 signal, and a "bright rim sign" on FLAIR imaging.

Discussion: DNETs are slow growing, benign, mixed glial-neuronal neoplasms. These are believed to originate from secondary germinal layer elements. These are usually centred on the cortical grey matter and large majority are associated with cortical dysplasia.

Over 60% are found in the temporal lobe, and 30% in the frontal lobe. These present with pharmacologically intractable partial complex seizures and 20-40% show enhancement.

Differential diagnosis:

   x   Ganglioglioma
   x   Pleomorphic xanthoastrocytoma (PXA)
   x   Diffuse low-grade astrocytoma
   x   Oligodendroglioma
   x   Desmoplastic infant astrocytomas and gangliogliomas

Case 9

Dr Timothy Ariyanayagam

A 3-year-old male presents with a frontal midline mass.

What is the diagnosis?

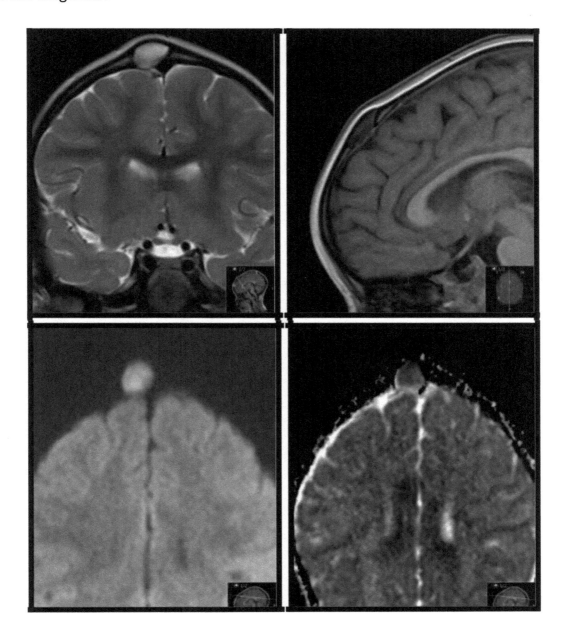

Intraosseous Epidermoid Cyst

Findings: Imaging reveals a well-defined T2-hyperintense lesion, which demonstrates restricted diffusion.

Discussion: Intracranial epidermoid cysts are inclusion cysts of ectodermal origin, consisting of keratinising squamous epithelium. Intradural epidermoids are likely caused by incomplete separation of neural and cutaneous ectoderm in the neural groove. Extradural intracranial epidermoids (roughly 10% of intracranial epidermoid cysts are extradural) are the result of trapping of cutaneous ectodermal remnants within cranial bones, or rarely traumatic implantation of squamous epithelium (this mechanism is more commonly seen in the phalanges as epidermal inclusion cysts).

These are of high T2 signal. They also have low T1 signal, which helps to differentiate intradural epidermoids from cholesterol containing dermoid cysts which show high T1 signal. They characteristically show restricted diffusion. Epidermoids also lack fat allowing differentiation from teratomas.

Case 10

Dr Timothy Ariyanayagam

A 3-month-old infant presents with a long, narrow head.

What is the diagnosis?

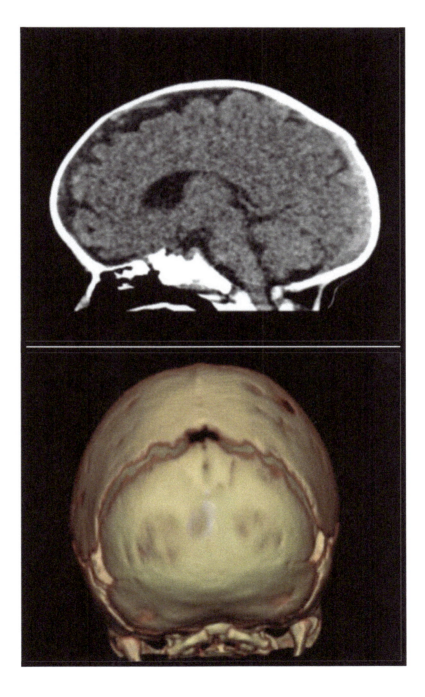

Craniosynostosis: Scaphocephaly

Findings: On the sagittal CT there is elongation of the skull in the AP direction. On the 3D reformats the sagittal suture is fused.

Discussion: Non-syndromic craniosynostosis refers to the premature closure of cranial sutures. This may be primary (considered to be premature fusion as a developmental error), or secondary (premature closure due to other factors such as intrauterine skull compression, teratogens or haematological conditions).

Syndromic craniosynostosis occurs in combination with craniofacial anomalies e.g. Apert Syndrome, Saethre-Chotzen syndrome or Pfeiffer Syndrome.

The subsequent pattern of head growth and shape is dependent on which suture(s) are fused. The diagnosis may be made on plain film, or CT with 3D reformats which allow better evaluation of the cranial sutures.

The commonest type of craniosynostosis is scaphocephaly. This is due to early closure of the sagittal suture, as demonstrated above on the 3D reformat, which prevents further lateral growth while allowing on-going AP growth. The result is a long, narrow skull.

- x Brachycephaly is due to bilateral coronal or lambdoid suture fusion resulting in a rounded skull shape.
- x Plagiocephaly is due to a unilateral coronal or lambdoid suture fusion, resulting in an asymmetrical skull shape.
- x Trigonocephaly is due to metopic suture fusion, resulting in a wedge-shaped skull.
- x Oxycephaly is due to bilateral closure of the coronal and lambdoid sutures, resulting in a "tower shaped" skull. This is one of the most severe craniosynostoses.

Kleeblattschädel, or clover-leaf skull, is a severe craniosynostosis resulting from closure of the coronal, lambdoid and sagittal sutures.

Case 11

Dr Timothy Ariyanayagam

A 5-year-old with developmental delay has been followed up regularly by the neurosurgical team.

Describe the abnormalities. What is the diagnosis?

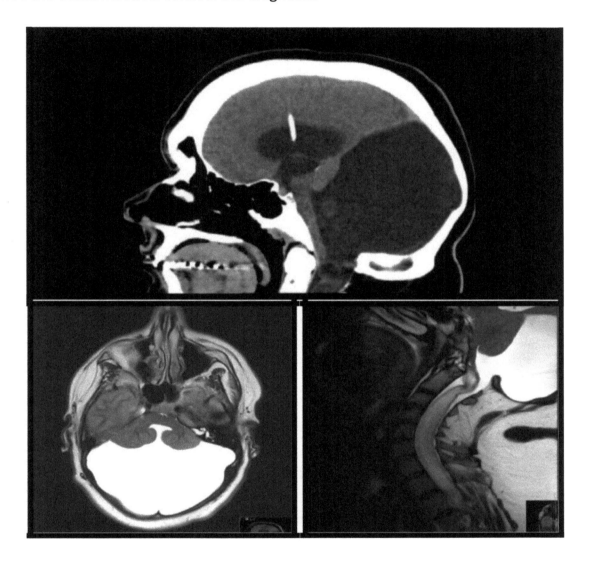

Dandy-Walker malformation with syrinx

Findings: There is an enlarged posterior fossa, a hypoplastic cerebellar vermis with cephalad rotation, and a cystic dilatation of the 4th ventricle (that fills nearly the entire enlarged posterior fossa). There is also hydrocephalus and a syringomyelia within the cervical spinal cord.

Discussion: The Dandy-Walker Complex/Continuum is a group of posterior fossa cystic malformations including the Dandy-Walker Malformation (DWM), Hypoplastic Vermis with Rotation (HVR) and Mega Cisterna Magna (MCM). Within this spectrum, the Dandy-Walker Malformation (DWM) is the "classical" form.

The key features are those found in the above case of a large posterior fossa, hypoplastic cerebellar vermis and cystic dilatation of the 4th ventricle. "Torcular-lamboid inversion" may also be seen in which the cyst prevents the usual descent of the torcular herophili. The patient will usually present with signs and symptoms of hydrocephalus by around 3 months of age (hydrocephalus is unusual at birth).

HVR is a milder form of cystic malformation. The key features are of a variable vermian hypoplasia and less cystic dilatation of the 4th ventricle than in classical DWM. Unlike in DWM, the posterior fossa is not enlarged. HVR replaces the term "Dandy-Walker Variant" which is confusing and somewhat archaic.

MCM consists of an enlarged cisterna magna causing enlargement of the posterior fossa, with a normal cerebellar vermis and 4th ventricle. One possible theory is that it results from delayed perforation of the Posterior Membranous Area.

The differential diagnosis for DWM includes a Blake's Pouch Cyst. Blake's pouch is a developmental cystic outpouching of the Posterior Membranous Area before it perforates to form the midline foramen of Magendie. If this outpouching persists, and fails to connect to the subarachnoid space, it forms a Blake's Pouch Cyst. The key features are of a cystic dilatation of the 4th ventricle, with a normal cerebellum and vermis. Some authors consider Blake's Pouch Cysts to be part of the Dandy-Walker Complex, but others argue that as it is not related to 4th ventricle and cerebellar malformations, it should be classified separately.

Case 12

Dr Timothy Ariyanayagam

A 3-month-old infant presents with "salaam attacks".

What are the abnormalities? What is the diagnosis?

What are the other intracranial manifestations of this disease? What are the diagnostic criteria?

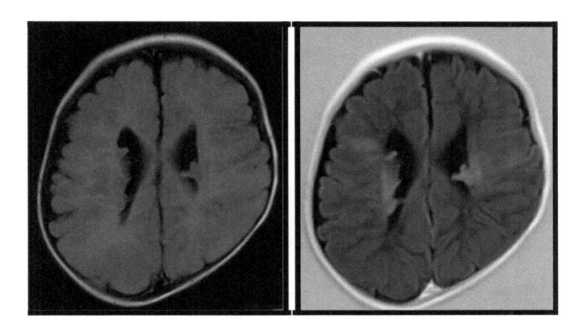

Tuberous Sclerosis

Findings: There are periventricular high FLAIR lesions and some high FLAIR lesions within the subcortical white matter. These are in keeping with subependymal and cortical tubers.

Discussion: The signal characteristics of these can be somewhat variable but are typically T1 hyperintense and T2/FLAIR iso- to hyper-intense, seen as subependymal nodules. These tend to calcify over time as the patient ages. These are associated with tuberous sclerosis.

Tuberous sclerosis is a congenital neurocutaneous syndrome. It may result from spontaneous mutation, or through autosomal dominant inheritance. It is characterised by a variety of hamartomatous lesions in multiple organs.

The other CNS abnormalities described in tuberous sclerosis include:

Cortical tubers – areas of loss of normal cortical layers, with dysmorphic giant cells and large astrocytes. These appear as cortical lesions with high T2 / low T1 signal. Histological evidence of these is pathognomonic of tuberous sclerosis.

Subependymal Giant Cell Astrocytoma (SEGA) – these are considered to be mixed glial-neuronal tumours of large cells that resemble astrocytes or glial cells; they are thought to arise from subependymal nodules. These tend to be larger (>1cm) than subependymal nodules and most often located near the foramen of Monroe, where these may cause obstructive hydrocephalus. When smaller, these cannot be reliably distinguished from subependymal nodules on imaging, except via serial scanning to demonstrate growth.

White matter abnormalities – these include the superficial white matter abnormalities that may be associated with cortical tubers, radial bands which are T2 hyper-intense, or cyst-like lesions.

Other extra-neuronal findings include renal angiomyolipomas, renal cysts, Shagreen patches, periungual fibromas, ash leaf macules, cardiac rhabdomyomas, and thoracic lymphangiomyomatosis.

Case 13

Dr Timothy Ariyanayagam

A 10-year-old child presents with a seizure. She is noted to have a left facial naevus flammeus in the trigeminal V_1 distribution.

What is the abnormality? What is the diagnosis?

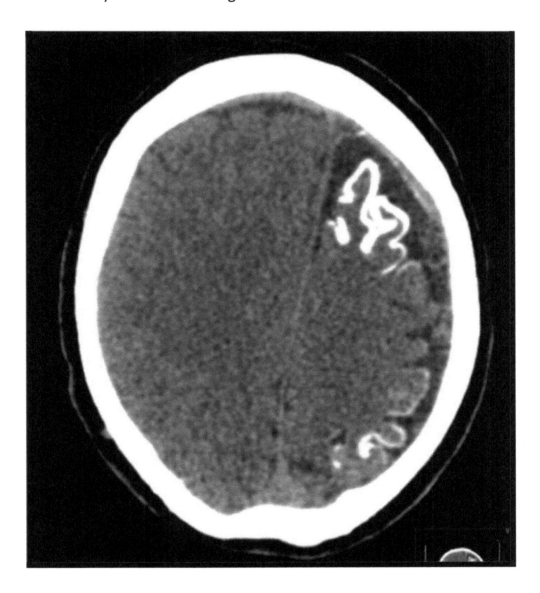

Sturge Weber Syndrome*

Findings: The CT slices above demonstrate "gyriform" subcortical and cortical calcification with atrophy of the left hemisphere.

Discussion: Sturge-Weber syndrome is a congenital neurocutaneous syndrome characterised by angiomatosis involving the face, choroid of the eye, and the leptomeninges.

The facial naevus flammeus, also known as a port wine stain, is often unilateral and most commonly in the V_1 trigeminal distribution. It is formed of multiple thin-walled blood vessels.

Intracranially, these are leptomeningeal angiomata. Calcification occurs in the adjacent brain, beginning subcortically and extending to involve the cortex.

Case 14

Dr Timothy Ariyanayagam

A 6-week-old infant presents as a floppy baby.

What is the abnormality? What are some common associations with this?

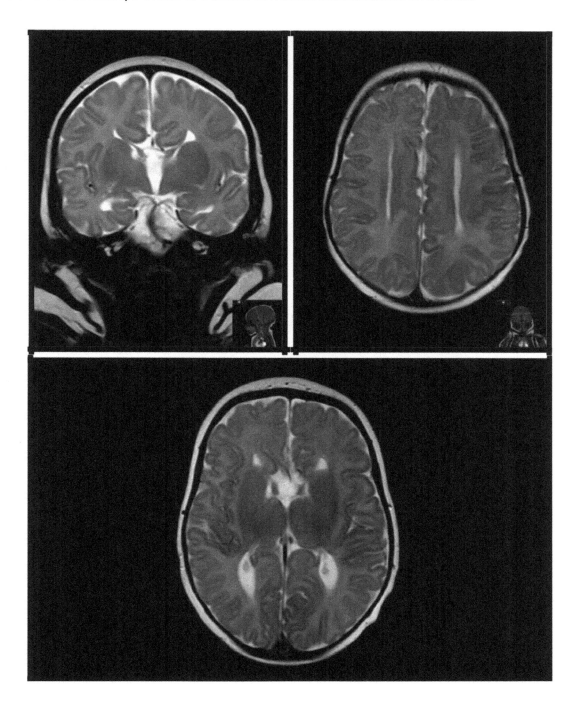

Agenesis of the Corpus Callosum

Findings: The images show widely spaced lateral ventricles, and a high-riding 3rd ventricle. The diagnosis was initially made on antenatal USS.

A scan of the same patient performed at 2 years of age shows the bundles of Probst between the widely spaced lateral ventricles:

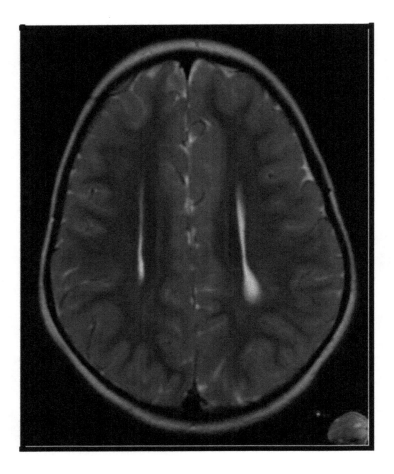

Discussion: Dysgenesis (complete or partial) of the corpus callosum may be associated with several conditions, including Edward's syndrome (trisomy 18), Patau syndrome (trisomy 13), Aicardi syndrome, Apert syndrome, Bickers-Adams-Edwards syndrome, Coffin-Siris syndrome, foetal alcohol syndrome, Fryns syndrome, Gorlin-Goltz syndrome, hydrolethalus syndrome, Lowe syndrome, and Zellweger syndrome.

Associated CNS abnormalities include Chiari II malformations, Dandy-Walker Complex, grey matter heterotopia, holoprosencephaly, hydrocephalus / colpocephaly, polymicrogyria, and porencephaly.

Case 15

Dr Timothy Ariyanayagam

A 7-year-old female involved in high speed RTA presents with GCS of 3/15

What is the abnormality? What are the consequences of this seen on the image?

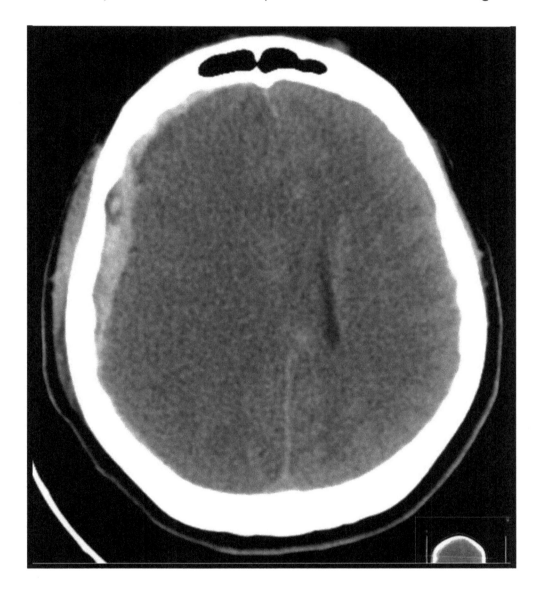

Subdural haemorrhage and midline shift

Findings: Imaging demonstrates a lentiform high density collection. There is also diffuse loss of the grey-white matter differentiation and swelling of the right hemisphere. This, along with the subdural haematoma, is causing a midline shift.

Discussion: Subdural haemorrhage may occur in any age group because of shearing of bridging veins crossing to drain into venous sinuses. In the paediatric age group, these are classically considered to raise the possibility of non-accidental injury (NAI), particularly in the context of a mixed density collection, and with concurrent signs such as retinal haemorrhages and encephalopathy. In this case, given the clear history and evidence of a high impact RTA, NAI is less of a concern.

In the above case there are areas of lower density seen as well, which is believed to represent a mixture of unclotted blood and serum in the "hyperacute" stage of injury before there has been time for homogeneous clot formation. Patients are rarely imaged during this stage.

Case 16

Dr Timothy Ariyanayagam

A 6-year-old child with known cerebral palsy is scanned.

What are the abnormalities? What is the probable diagnosis? Are the imaging features specific?

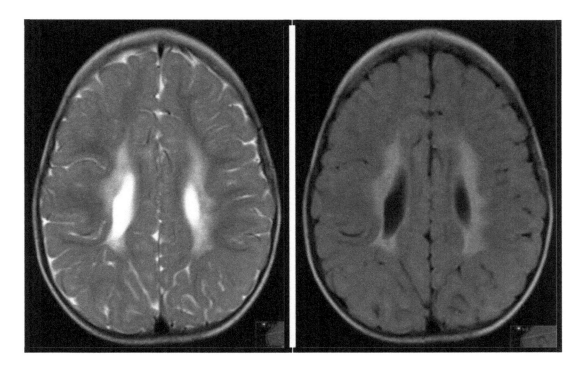

White matter disease of prematurity – longstanding

Findings: The images above demonstrate periventricular white matter T2/FLAIR hyperintensity, with marked loss of white matter volume. There is irregularity of the ventricles, suggestive of some ex vacuo dilatation.

Discussion: White matter disease of prematurity (previously called periventricular leukomalacia) ... these features are non-specific, and could be due to a variety of causes, including ventriculitis, inborn errors of metabolism or hydrocephalus. In the context of a patient with known hypoxic-ischaemic brain injury and resultant cerebral palsy, these features are likely to represent any of the following:

Hypoxic-Ischaemic brain injury in a neonate can have different imaging pattern manifestations depending upon several factors, such as whether the neonate is term or pre-term, the severity of hypotension, and the duration of hypotension.

In the pre-term infant, with mild to moderate hypotension, the injury tends to be limited to the periventricular white matter. This is postulated to be due to supply to this area being from peripheral penetrating vessels, with poorly formed or absent ventriculofugal vessels. As the brain matures, the watershed area that becomes injured with hypotension moves peripherally.

Acutely, there is T2 hyperintensity in the periventricular white matter with smaller areas of T1 hyperintensity seen within. As this injury matures there is necrosis and cavitation with the formation of multiple small cysts. These cysts often decrease in size over time and can disappear.

The appearances of end-stage PVL on MRI include periventricular white matter T2 hyperintensity, loss of white matter volume, and ex vacuo dilatation of the ventricles.

Case 17

Dr Timothy Ariyanayagam

This 11-year-old male presents with an ascending paralysis. There is a history of a diarrhea of recent origin

Describe the abnormality on the T1 and T1 + contrast weighted sagittal images. What is the diagnosis?

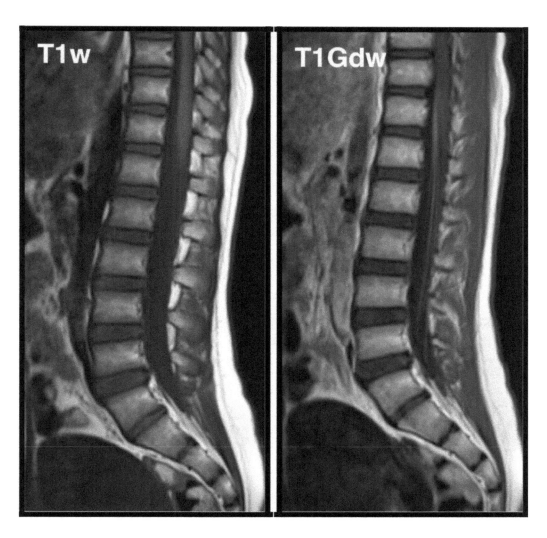

Guillain-Barre Syndrome

Findings: The images above show marked enhancement of the cauda equina and the post-contrast T1 weighted images.

Discussion: Cauda equina enhancement has a wide general differential (e.g. AIDS polyradiculopathy, arachnoiditis, neurosarcoidosis, leptomeningeal carcinomatosis, chronic inflammatory demyelinating polyneuropathy, Lyme disease or rabies), but in this clinical context, is in keeping with Guillain-Barré syndrome (GBS).

GBS is an inflammatory, peripheral polyradiculoneuropathy. It is often preceded by an upper respiratory tract infection or diarrheal illness (in particular, Campylobacter jejuni) a few weeks prior to onset; the aetiology is believed to be autoimmune with molecular mimicry of certain pathogenic gangliosides resulting in damage to axons or demyelination. There are several subtypes, including acute inflammatory demyelinating polyradiculoneuropathy (AIDP), acute motor axonal neuropathy (AMAN), acute motor sensory axonal neuropathy (AMSAN), or regional subtypes such as the Miller-Fisher variant.

The classical clinical presentation is of a symmetrical, ascending flaccid paresis with variable sensory or autonomic involvement. It is a self-limiting disorder but can result in respiratory failure.

The diagnosis is often made with a combination of clinical examination and history, CSF biochemistry, and nerve conduction studies. Imaging may also be helpful, but it is important to give contrast as the unenhanced appearances are essentially normal.

Case 18

Dr Sarah Abdulla

An 8-year-old child presents with frontal headaches and vomiting for 5 days. What is the examination and what are your findings?

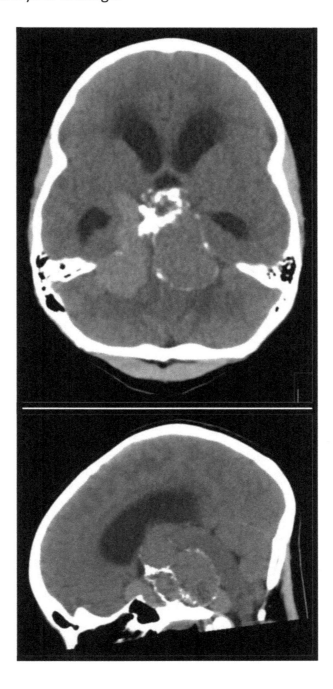

Craniopharyngioma

Findings: There is a large soft tissue and calcified lesion in the suprasellar and pre-pontine cisterns. The mass is compressing the brainstem and causing hydrocephalus of the lateral ventricles.

Discussion: Craniopharyngiomas are low-grade, suprasellar mass lesions that have a bimodal age distribution. Those occurring in the paediatric population are mostly the adamantinomatous subtype which have multiple cysts filled with an oily fluid containing protein, blood and/or cholesterol. There may be a few soft tissue foci that enhance, and calcification is very common.

They can be very large and cause mass effect and hydrocephalus, which will present as a headache, visual disturbances and hormonal imbalance due to the close proximity of the optic chiasm and pituitary gland.

Treatment is with surgical resection with radiotherapy for residual disease.

Benign recurrence can be seen in up to 30% of cases.

Differential diagnosis:

- x Pituitary adenoma
- x Rathke's cleft cyst
- x Teratoma

Case 19

Dr Gema Priego

A 2-year-old boy with polydactyly was found to have an intracranial mass.

Where is the epicentre of the abnormality? Is there any syndrome associated?

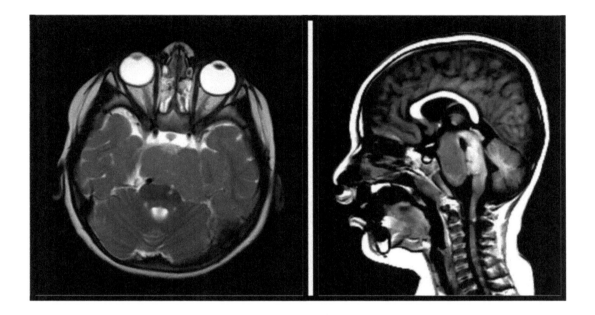

Hall Syndrome

Findings: There is an enlarged mass centred in the hypothalamus. The lesion causes severe mass effect upon optic chiasm and third ventricle, resulting in mild hydrocephalus. There is also marked mass effect upon the pituitary, which can result in a wide symptomatology from panhypopituitarism to asymptomatic patients. The lesion is isointense to the grey matter on T1wi and T2wi, with no enhancement and no evidence of calcification on a CT. Findings were consistent with a giant hamartoma. The MRI findings makes unlikely other suprasellar tumours, such as: Craniopharyngioma (enhancement and calcifications) and macroadenoma (T1-hypointense, T2-hyperintense and far less common in paediatrics).

Discussion: The size of this hamartoma is very characteristic of Pallister-Hall Syndrome, which is also associated to other major anomalies: polydactyly, cutaneous syndactyly, bifid epiglottis, anal atresia and genitourinary malformations (cryptorchidism, renal hypoplasia or agenesis and renal ectopia).

The patient was confirmed with a GLI3 gene mutation on chromosome 7p13. Pallister-Hall syndrome is an important diagnosis for future genetic counselling, to look for associated anomalies and to screen asymptomatic parents for hypothalamic hamartomas with brain MR imaging

Clinical management of these patients will include endocrinologic assessment for panhypopituitarism, visual-field ophthalmologic assessment, follow brain MR imaging for tumour progression, and a dedicated search for previously mentioned anomalies.

1. Biesecker LG. Pallister-Hall Syndrome. Gene Reviews. NCBI.
2. Kuo Js, Casey SO, Thompson L and Truwit L. AJNR 1999, 20(10) 1839-41

Head and neck cases

Case 1

Dr Timothy Ariyanayagam

An 8-year-old male presents with conductive hearing loss.

What is the imaging abnormality?

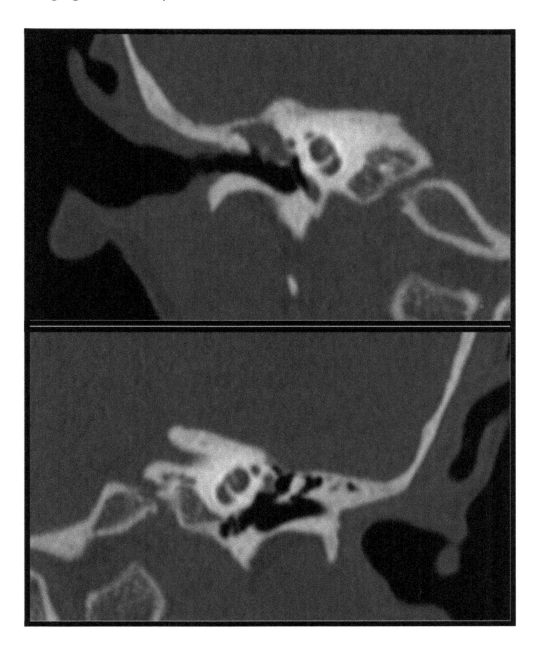

Cholesteatoma

Findings: The first coronal CT image shows soft tissue density material within the right epitympanum and mesotympanum, with erosion of the malleus and incus. The second image shows the normal contralateral left side.

Discussion: Cholesteatomas are non-neoplastic abnormal growths of keratinising squamous epithelium.

Congenital cholesteatomas are rare and represent extra-dural, intra-osseous, ectodermal inclusions; these are histologically equivalent to intracranial epidermoid cysts, which are intra-dural ectodermal inclusions. These tend to occur in the petrous apex or, if found in the middle ear, around the head of the malleus and body of incus.

Acquired cholesteatomas are more common. There are several hypotheses regarding their aetiology. It is possible that these form due to Eustachian tube dysfunction and tympanic membrane retraction, migration of keratinising cells through a perforation, basal cell hyperplasia of the tympanic membrane secondary to infection, metaplasia from chronic infection, or possibly a combination of all these. Acquired cholesteatomas can arise from the pars tensa or the pars flaccida.

Case 2

Dr Sarah Abdulla

A 9-year-old female presents with congenital sensorineural hearing loss.

What is the imaging abnormality?

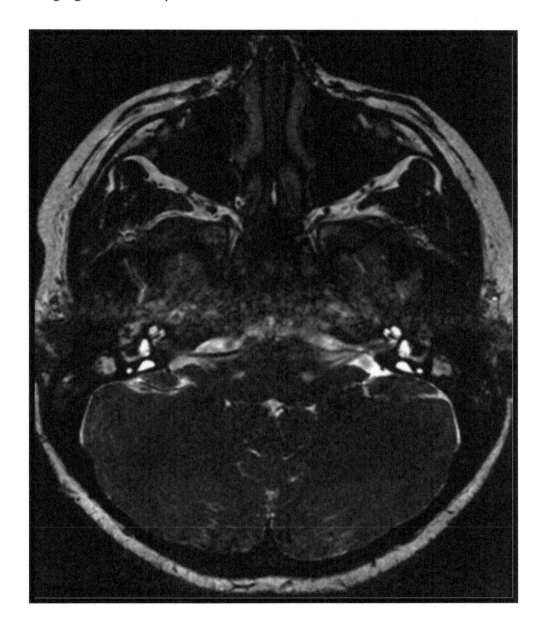

Case 2

Large vestibular aqueduct syndrome

Findings: On the T2-CISS sequence slices the vestibular aqueducts are enlarged bilaterally measuring 2.5mm.

Discussion: Large vestibular aqueduct syndrome (LVAS) is thought to be one of the most common causes of congenital sensorineural hearing loss although hearing loss is not inevitable in all patients. The usual upper limit of the normal vestibular aqueduct is 1.5mm in AP dimension at the mid-point between the crus commune and external aperture.

There are associated anomalies in up to 85% of patients including Pendred syndrome and vestibular, cochlear, and semicircular canal anomalies.

Case 3

Dr Khalid Khan

A 13-year-old presents with worsening right periorbital cellulitis and a persistent fever.

What is this examination and what are your findings?

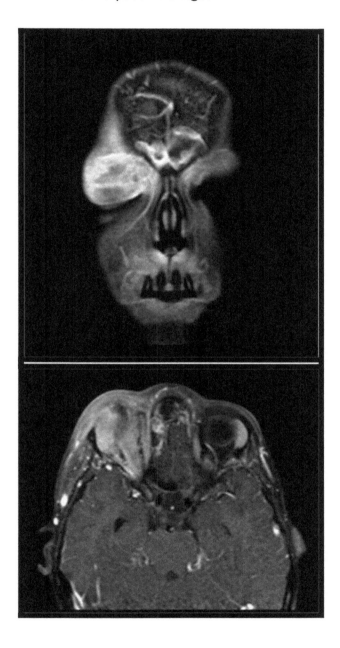

Orbital cellulitis

Findings: On these fat saturated T1 weighted contrast-enhanced MRI images of the orbits there is soft tissue swelling overlying the right orbit, which extends to involve the intraorbital fat. The findings are in keeping with pre- and post-septal orbital cellulitis.

Discussion: Orbital infection is common in the paediatric population. The most common causes are spread via the sinuses, face or teeth.

If the infection is limited to the soft tissue anterior to the orbital septum (pre-septal cellulitis) it can be managed with oral antibiotics. If, however, the infection extends into the orbit (post-septal cellulitis) this is more serious and requires hospitalisation and parenteral antibiotics. It is important to look for any complications such as intraorbital abscess formation (as in this case) as these require surgical drainage.

The complications of orbital cellulitis include:

- x   Superior ophthalmic vein and cavernous sinus thrombosis
- x   Loss of vision
- x   Intracranial spread with subdural empyema, meningitis and intracranial abscess

Case 4

Dr Khalid Khan

A 12-year-old boy with sickle cell disease presents with neck stiffness and pyrexia with a palpable neck mass.

What are these examinations and what are your findings?

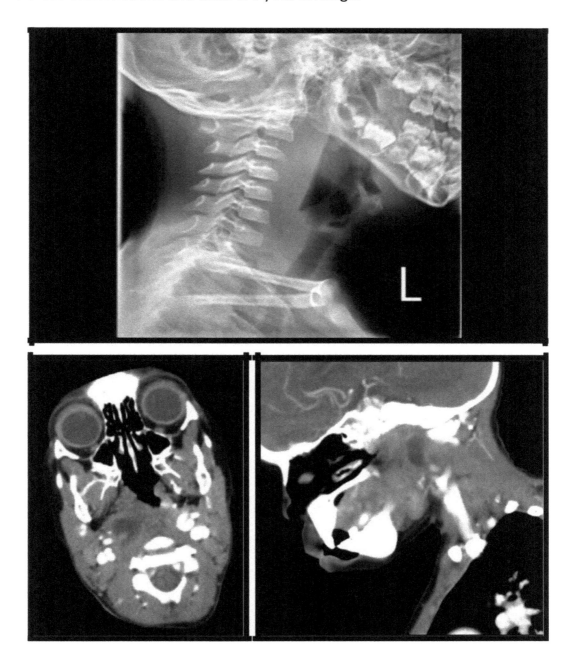

Retropharyngeal abscess

Finding: On the radiograph there is marked thickening of the soft tissues in the prevertebral space extending from C2-C7. On the post-contrast CT images there is a hypodense area in the right retropharyngeal region with peripheral enhancement in keeping with a retropharyngeal abscess.

Discussion: Retropharyngeal abscesses are life-threatening infections. These can progress to cause respiratory compromise. These can also spread inferiorly into the mediastinum, posteriorly into the vertebrae and spinal canal and laterally into the carotid space to cause jugular vein thrombosis.

In the paediatric population retropharyngeal abscesses are usually due to spread of infection from the upper respiratory tract. Less commonly penetrating injuries, such as ingestion of foreign objects, may cause infection due to penetration.

The most common causative organisms are β -haemolytic streptococci and *Staphylococcus aureus*. On radiographs there may be prevertebral soft tissue swelling. The normal thickness of soft tissue at the level of the C2 vertebra is less than 7 mm. At the C6 level a good rule of thumb is that the soft tissue should be less than ½ the width of the vertebral body. In children younger than 15 years old this corresponds to 14 mms

Case 5

Dr Khalid Khan

A 10-year-old male presents with a long-standing midline neck lump that moves on tongue protrusion.

What is the diagnosis?

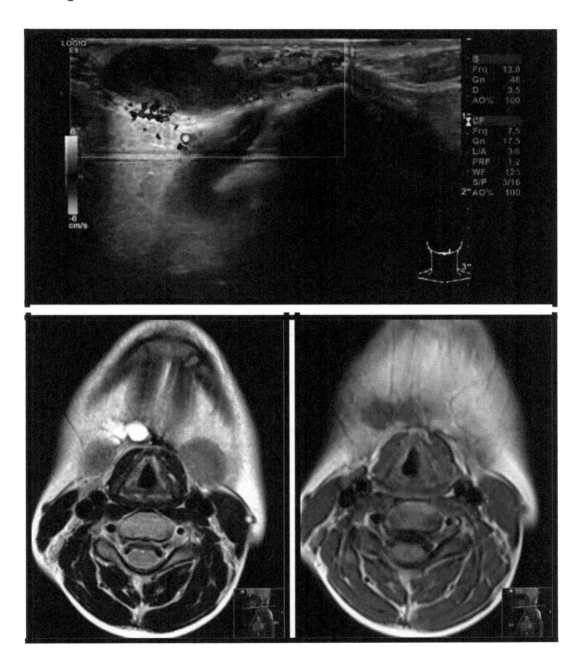

Thyroglossal duct cyst

Findings: The ultrasound imaging above reveals a lobulated, debris-filled cystic lesion in the right sub-mental region. This is also seen on the axial MRI slices. In this case, these actually represent a Thyroglossal cyst remnant, from a previous operation 2 years ago.

Discussion: Thyroglossal duct cysts represent a fluid filled remnant of the thyroglossal duct and they are a common cause of a neck mass in children. As such, these may be found in the midline at any point from the foramen caecum at the base of the tongue, to the level of the thyroid gland. These commonly move with swallowing and elevate on tongue protrusion.

They are usually asymptomatic until they become infected.

On imaging these do not enhance and usually are proteinaceous or may show previous haemorrhage or infection.

Case 6a

Dr Khalid Khan

A 6-year-old male presents with multiple lumps in the neck on both sides. There is a recent history of sore throat.

What is this examination and what does it show?

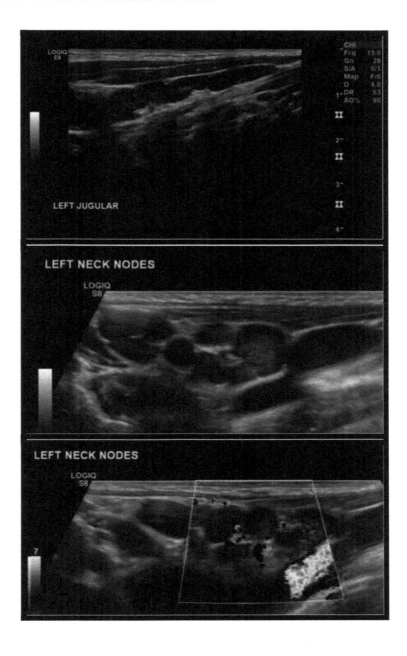

Case 6b

Another patient presents with a recent history of throat infection and now has a swelling in the left submandibular area.

What are these examinations and what do they show?

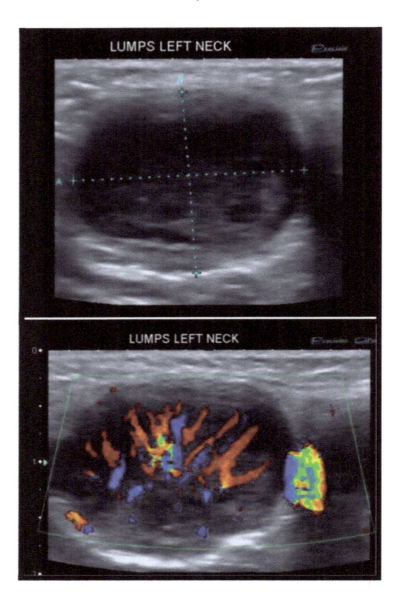

Benign neck lymphadenopathy

Findings case 6a: This ultrasound examination shows several enlarged lymph nodes in the soft tissues of the left posterior auricular region, carotid chains bilaterally and posterior chains. The lymph nodes have no internal vascularity.

Findings case 6b: The ultrasound shows a well-defined solid lesion noted in the left submandibular gland, which demonstrates increased vascularity on Doppler.

Discussion: Cervical lymphadenopathy is commonly seen in children who have had a recent history of ear, nose, or throat infection. The child usually presents with a painful mass in the neck.

There are multiple chains of lymph nodes seen in the soft tissues of the anterior and posterior part of the neck. The superficial lymph nodes that can be identified on ultrasound are commonly encountered in the posterior auricular area, along the carotid jugular complex, in the submental and submandibular areas. Lymphadenopathy in supraclavicular area should be viewed with suspicion

Lymph nodes can also be seen in relation to the salivary glands such as the parotid and submandibular gland. Normal lymph nodes are far more numerous in younger individuals and one may find the 10-20 nodes in an asymptomatic patient.

Lymph nodes on ultrasound are typically oval structures measuring 0.1 - 2.5 cm long. Normal benign lymph node is an elliptical structure with an outer hypoechoic cortex and a central bright echogenic hilum. The echogenic hilum represents fat within the node. On Doppler, a blood vessel is usually seen to enter at the hilum.

Lymph nodes up to 3-4 cm in length are often seen in normal individuals particularly children. Multiple lymph nodes are sometimes matted together to form a large mass. It then becomes difficult to assess the size of an individual node.

The grey-scale parameters that favour malignancy

1. Size: Larger - more likely malignant
2. Shape: elliptical benign and a rounded shape of the lymph node favours malignancy
3. Heterogeneous echo texture
4. Loss of central fatty hilum/thinning of hilum
5. Eccentric/concentric thickening of cortex and a spiculated margin
6. Micro calcification
7. Necrosis - cystic/coagulative
8. Ill-defined capsular margins suggestive of invasion

Colour Doppler features that favour malignancy

1. Peripheral blood vessels
2. Curved course of intranodal vessels
3. Focal absence of perfusion
4. Subcapsular vessels that do not originate from the hilum
5. High resistance wave form
6. RI>.8, PI>1.5
7. Aberrant vessels – displaced parent vessels, subcapsular vasculature, unperfused areas, non-tapering vessels

When Malignancy is suspected excisional biopsy is suggested.

Case 7

Dr Khalid Khan

A 7-year-old child presents with a recent history of an enlarged parotid glands and fever.

What is the examination and what are your findings?

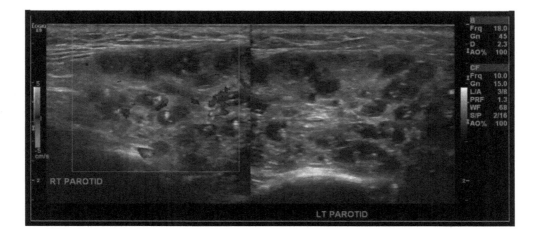

Parotitis

Findings: The ultrasound of both parotid glands shows enlarged parotid glands with multiple areas of low echogenicity and increased vascularity.

Discussion: Parotitis in children is uncommon. The most common cause in the paediatric population is viral, in particular mumps. Other causes include suppurative parotitis secondary to a bacterial infection, which may develop into an abscess. In some, no cause is found, such as in recurrent parotitis of childhood.

Patients usually present with anorexia, headache, fever and malaise.

On ultrasound the parotid glands are enlarged and heterogeneous. There may be some enlarged intra-parotid lymph nodes evident and increased vascularity of the affected gland. Mumps may involve other organs such as the pancreas, the meninges and, in males, testes.

Musculoskeletal cases

Case 1

Dr Trevor Gaunt and Dr Gema Priego

Newborn is presenting with multiple dysmorphic features. Antenatal scan showed ventriculomegaly and narrow thoracic cage. Images below are provided from a skeletal survey.

What is the main abnormality in the skull? What is the main finding of the upper arm?

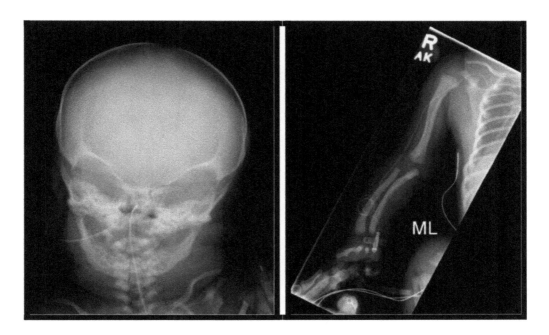

Shprintzen-Goldberg syndrome

Findings: Frontal radiograph of the skull shows premature fusion of both coronal sutures resulting in brachiocephaly. In addition, this causes elevation of the bilateral superior lateral corner of both orbits (harlequin eye deformity sign). The sagittal suture remains open.

The second radiograph of the right upper limbs shows bowing deformity of the long bones, mildly undermodelled. The bony density is maintained, and no pathological fracture seen. The ribs appear thin and slightly twisted. These findings may resemble those of frontometaphyseal dysplasia. However, the combination with craniosynostosis and the clinical history of ventriculomegaly is characteristic of Shprintzen Goldberg syndrome.

Discussion: Shprintzen-Goldberg syndrome (SGS) is a genetic disorder with a multisystem involvement. It is caused by a mutation in SKI gene, which contains a protein with an important role in development of many tissues including skin, brain and bones. Most of the cases are de novo mutations and sometimes other genes may be affected in this syndrome.

The major sign of SGS are craniosynostosis, skeletal findings are visible on the radiographs, cardiovascular findings (mitral or aortic regurgitation or mitral prolapse). Neurological symptoms are also striking with delayed motor and cognitive development and abnormal neuroimaging with ventriculomegaly and volume loss of the brain.

1. Greally MT. Shprintzen Goldberg syndrome. Gene Reviews. 2006.
2. Nishimura G, Nagai T. Radiographic findings in Shprintzen-Goldberg Syndrome. Pediatric Radiol. 1996; 26 (11): 775-8

Case 2

Dr Trevor Gaunt and Dr Khalid Khan

An 11-year-old presents with a recent history of vague pain in his left hip.

There is no history of trauma.

What are these examinations and what are your findings?

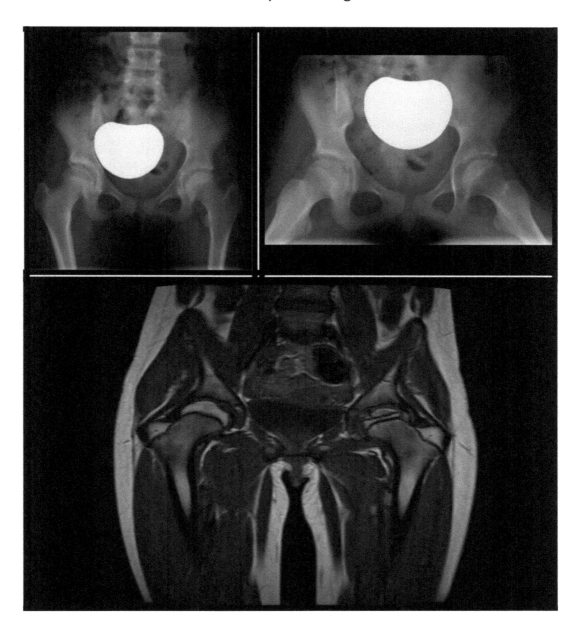

Perthes disease

Findings: On the plain film there is a small, flattened, sclerotic left proximal epiphysis. On the T1 weighted MRI the left epiphysis is smaller in volume and there is a fracture line through it.

Discussion: Perthe's disease (also referred to as Legg-Calvé-Perthe's disease) is avascular necrosis of the femoral head. The aetiology is unknown and it is generally accepted to be idiopathic. The peak incidence is around 5 to 6 years, but it can occur from 2 to 12 years old. It is five times more common in males.

15% of cases may be bilateral. Early in the process there may be no radiographical findings apart from subtle mottling of the affected femoral head and relative proximal metaphyseal blurring.

Later, there is subcortical crescentic lucency (crescent sign) which progresses to femoral head fragmentation and collapse. In advanced Perthe's disease there is widening and flatting of the femoral head (coxa plana). The femoral neck becomes widened to compensate for the changes in weight bearing leading to a coxa magna deformity.

MRI is now routinely used for early diagnosis and prognostication.

Differential diagnosis:

- x   Slipped upper femoral epiphysis
- x   Osteomyelitis
- x   Avascular necrosis of other cause
- x   Juvenile idiopathic arthritis
- x   Dysplasia epiphyseal capris femoris

Case 3

Dr Trevor Gaunt and Dr Khalid Khan

A term baby presents with a left axillary mass which is mobile and non-tender.

What are these examinations and what are your findings?

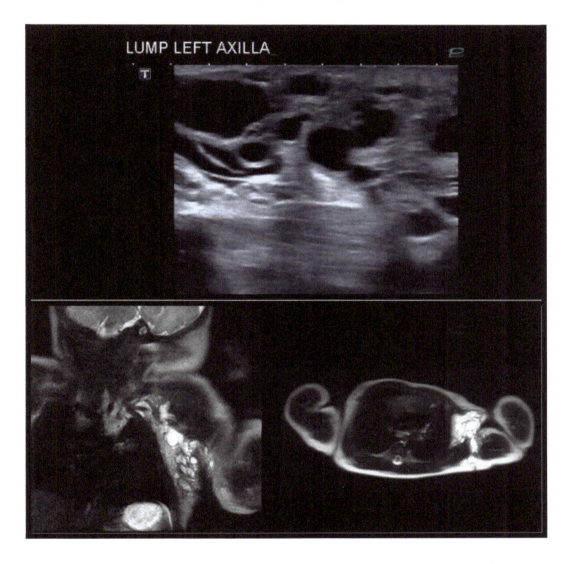

Cystic lymphangioma

Findings: On ultrasound there is a multicystic mass within the axilla. This was confirmed on MRI, which found a multicystic mass extending from the axilla along the lateral and anterior left chest wall.

Discussion: Cystic lymphangioma is a benign vascular lesion that is the lymphatic equivalent of haemangioma of blood vessels. These present at any age but is more common in children under 2-years-old. These may be associated with lymphangiomyomatosis.

These are a type of congenital lymphangioma that result from maldevelopment of the lymphatic system connection with the venous system.

The vast majority are in the head, neck and axillary regions although they may also be found in the liver, spleen, kidneys, retro peritoneum, lungs and mediastinum

On imaging these are cystic masses. These may become heterogeneous in appearance in the presence of proteinaceous fluid, internal haemorrhage or lipid components. In general, there is minimal displacement of adjacent structures unless there is rapid growth secondary to haemorrhage.

Associated anomalies are common particularly aneuploidic syndromes such as Turner, Down and trisomy 18, 13 and 11. There are also non-aneuploidic anomalies such as congenital heart disease, Apert syndrome, Cornelia de Lange syndrome and fetal alcohol syndrome.

Differential diagnosis:

   x   Venous malformation

Case 4

Dr Trevor Gaunt and Dr Khalid Khan

A 4-year-old presents with painless lump superficial to the left gastrocnemius.

What is the examination and what are your findings?

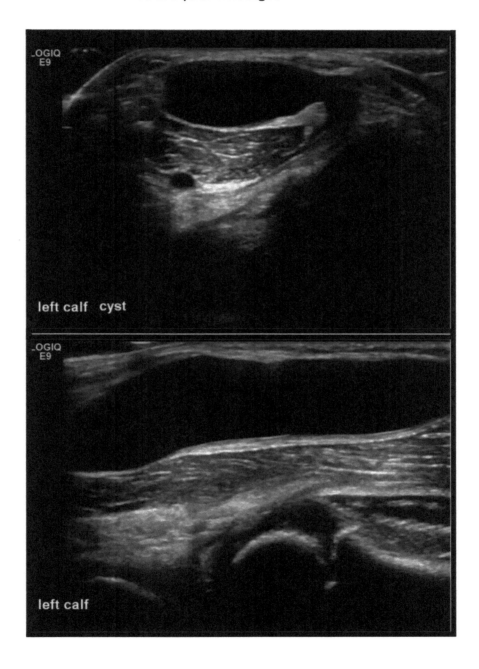

Baker's cyst

Findings: There is a well-defined simple cyst within the left popliteal fossa and calf, which is superficial to the muscles.

Discussion: Baker's cysts are fluid filled bursae with a synovial lining situated in the popliteal fossa. There is a bimodal age distribution with peaks at 4 to 7 years old and 35 to 70 years old.

Presentation may be with a mass or with a complication such as dissection with or without inter-muscular dissection, compression of the popliteal vessels or nerve and compartment syndrome. These can also rupture in which case these may present with symptoms of acute deep vein thrombosis.

Ultrasound shows a well-defined cyst between the medial head of gastrocnemius and semimembranosus tendons. Identification of the neck extending into the joint space is diagnostic. These are typically anechoic but may contain internal debris.

In children, most will spontaneously resolve within two years of presentation. Aspiration with steroid injection can be used to reduce the size and improve symptoms. Surgical excision may be necessary if symptoms persist or the cyst is very large.

Differential diagnosis:

x   Large Para meniscal cyst
x   Liquefied popliteal fossa haematoma

Case 5

Dr Khalid Khan

A 14-year-old boy presents with swelling over his right shoulder for 2 months, which is now painful.

What are these examinations and what are your findings?

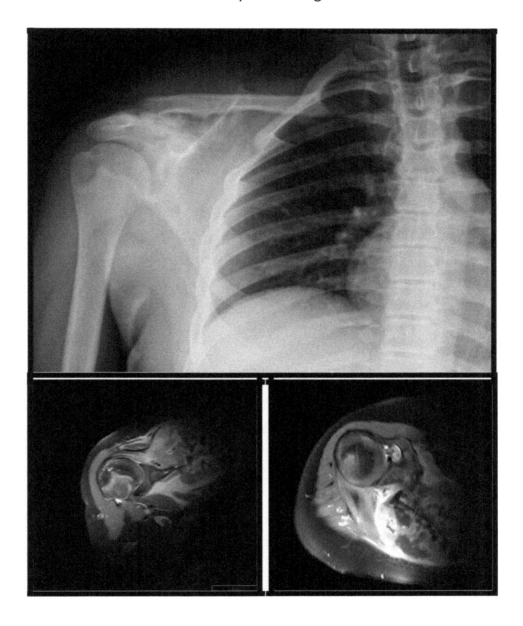

Ewing's sarcoma

Findings: on the shoulder radiograph there is a supraclavicular soft tissue mass and irregularity of the superior border of the scapula. On MRI this is a large heterogeneous enhancing soft tissue mass centred on the scapula, which is causing bony destruction. The bone scan shows high uptake in the lesion (image not given).

Discussion: Ewing's sarcoma is the second most common malignant paediatric primary bone tumour following osteosarcoma. The typical age range is 4 to 25 years old with a peak from 10 to 20 years old with a slight male predominance. These are small round blue cell tumour closely related to PNET, Askin tumours and neuroepitheliomas.

Presentation is usually non-specific with pain being the most common. There may also be a pathological fracture following trivial trauma. Patients can have systemic features with a low-grade fever and non-specifically raised inflammatory markers.

The most common location is the lower limb with the majority being found in the femur. The upper limb and axial skeleton are less commonly involved. Long bones are affected more commonly than flat bones and most are located centrally within the metadiaphysis or diaphysis.

Imaging shows highly aggressive features with a permeative, lytic abnormality and a lamellated periosteal reaction with a poorly defined margin. In very aggressive tumours there may be a more spiculated or sunburst type of periosteal reaction with Codman triangle. On MRI the mass is heterogeneous with foci of haemorrhage and avid, but heterogeneous, enhancement.

Staging requires nuclear medicine scan of the entire skeleton to identify bone metastasis and a CT thorax is recommended for identification of lung metastasis. Discussion with a regional bone tumour centre is necessary for referral for biopsy.

Differential diagnosis:

- x Osteosarcoma
- x Osteomyelitis
- x Langerhans cell histiocytosis

Case 6

Dr Khalid Khan

A 1-year-old child is brought into the emergency department unconscious.

The infant rolled over from the bed and has not regained consciousness.

The infant resuscitated, stabilized and later discharged home.

The patient had a skeletal survey. The chest radiographs did not show any pathology.

Two weeks later the patient had a cardiac arrest at home and the ambulance was called. Another skeletal survey was performed with the oblique chest radiograph displayed below. What are your findings?

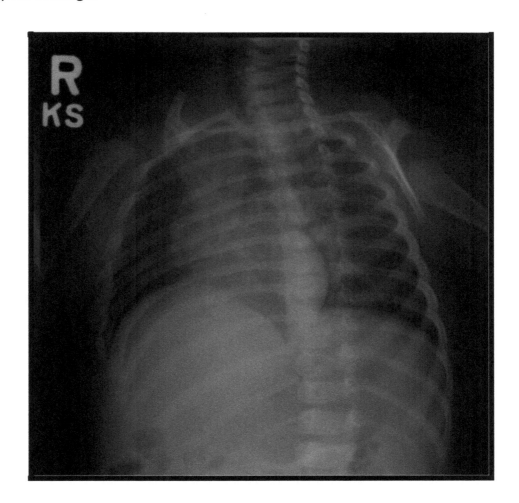

Non-accidental injury

Findings: on the initial skeletal survey there were no fractures demonstrated and the lungs were clear. On the repeat skeletal survey two weeks after there is a healing fracture of the posterior aspect of the right sixth rib.

Discussion: A 2011 literature review found that the most common perpetrator was the caregiver or parent, another relative, or a person in a relationship with the child's caregiver.

There are particular suspicious clinical features that should raise the alarm for NAI.

- x Injury in a non-ambulatory child
- x Incompatible injury and history
- x Delay in seeking medical attention
- x Multiple fractures which may be at different stages of healing in the absence of osteogenesis imperfecta or other metabolic bone diseases
- x Retinal haemorrhage
- x Torn frenulum

There are very specific guidelines to the imaging of suspected NAI in the UK which is available on the Royal College of Radiologists website. A skeletal survey must be performed by a trained radiographer and reported by two trained radiologists. There is a specific set of images that must be obtained.

Imaging features that are suspicious of NAI include:

- x Metaphyseal corner fractures / bucket handle fractures
- x Rib fractures, particularly posteriorly and at the costochondral junction
- x Skull fractures that involve multiple bones that cross sutures or are depressed or there is presence of diastatic sutures
- x Scapula, sternal, clavicular and first rib fractures in the absence of appropriate trauma

Differential Diagnosis

- x Osteogenesis imperfecta
- x Rickets
- x Birth injuries

Case 7

Dr Trevor Gaunt and Dr Khalid Khan Dr Faisal Alyas

A 16-year-old presented with sepsis, a cough and a painful left knee. On further questioning they had a 1-year history of difficulty in flexing the left knee.

What are these examinations and what are your findings?

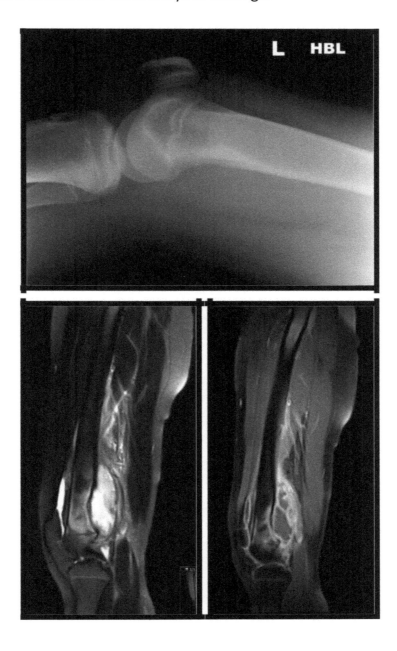

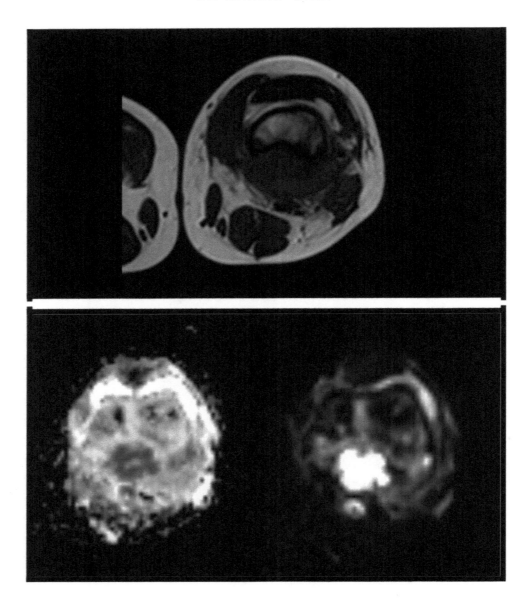

Subperiosteal tuberculous abscess

Findings: The radiograph shows a soft tissue swelling in the popliteal fossa. There is also subtle sclerosis and cortical irregularity of the metaphysis. The MRI confirms the cortical thickening and irregularity and shows a peripherally enhancing collection within the popliteal fossa with oedema of the adjacent femur. The collection shows restricted diffusion in keeping with a soft tissue abscess and associated osteomyelitis. An aspirate showed that this was a tuberculous abscess.

Discussion: Tuberculous abscess are most common between 2 and 12 years old with a 3:1 male preponderance.

Presentation is often non-specific with symptoms such as fever, rigors, lethargy and irritability. The classic signs of inflammation such as pain, swelling and erythema occurs in the acute setting but is mostly transient and may resolve after 5 to 7 days. On examination the patient may have a reduced range of movement, signs of trauma and oedema.

In most instances osteomyelitis results from haematogenous spread or via direct inoculation via trauma with the majority of infections due to *Staphylococcus aureus*. Tuberculous osteomyelitis is commonly due to haematogenous spread to the synovium.

The most common site of infection is the metaphysis of growing appendicular bones although a subperiosteal abscess can develop as in this case. This is likely due to the sharp angulation of arterioles feeding into venous sinusoids and a relative lack of regional macrophages.

The earliest sign on radiography is a loss or blurring of normal fat planes. However, skeletal changes are only apparent after at least a 30% loss of bone mineral content. Regional osteopenia, endosteal scalloping and loss of bone architecture are common findings. Periosteal reaction is a non-specific finding but may suggest chronicity or a subperiosteal abscess as in this case. A Brodie's abscess commonly appears as a well-defined, round lucency which crosses the physis.

On MRI acute osteomyelitis demonstrate low T1 and high T2 bone marrow signal with ill-defined margins and avid enhancement. Non-enhancing areas are likely to be due to necrosis.

On plain film chronic osteomyelitis may show a thick periosteal reaction with a well-defined region of sclerotic, necrotic bone within the bony medulla (sequestrum). An opening into the soft tissues may be seen from the involucrum, known as a cloaca. On MRI there low T1 and T2 signal due to fibrosis and sclerosis with regions of cortical thickening.

Differential diagnosis:

- x   Langerhans cell histiocytosis
- x   Ewing's sarcoma
- x   Paraosteal osteosarcoma

Case 8

Dr Trevor Gaunt and Dr Khalid Khan Dr Faisal Alyas

A 15-year-old female presented with a swelling in the anterior right ankle that has been getting bigger gradually and is now causing pain.

What are these examinations and what are your findings?

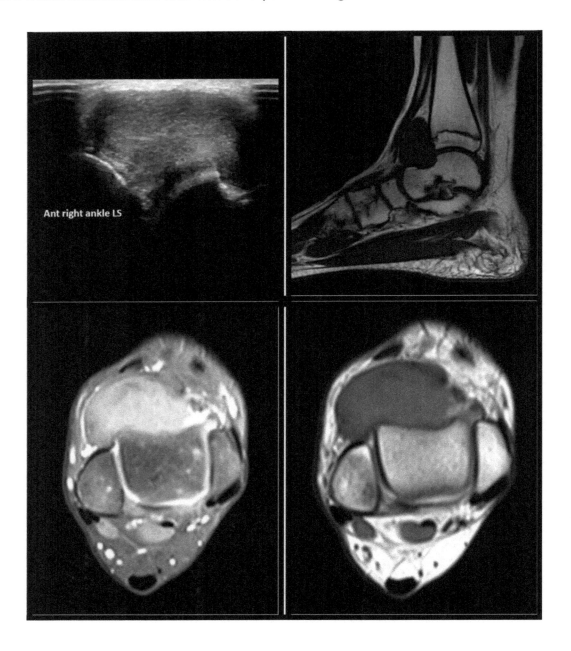

Synovial sarcoma

Findings: On ultrasound there is a soft tissue mass in the anterior ankle joint space with no internal vascularity. On MRI this lesion has low T1 signal with homogeneous enhancement, which is closely related to the anterior ankle joint.

Discussion: Synovial sarcomas most commonly present in adolescents and young adults with a peak age of 15-40 years old with a mild male predilection.

The term "synovial" refers to the fact that the cells resemble normal synovial cells, but they express different epithelial markers to normal synovium. These are commonly located around a large joint but do not arise from the synovium itself. The most common locations are in the extremities with the lower limb more frequently involved than the upper limb. Other sites include the pharynx, conjunctiva and nervous system. Rarely these may involve the chest wall and abdominal viscera.

On plain radiography bony involvement is well demonstrated with benign-appearing bony erosion or more aggressive features such as periosteal reaction or a permeative, moth-eaten appearance. Ultrasound shows non-specific features of a heterogeneous mass. On CT the mass is of mixed attenuation with heterogeneous enhancement. Calcification and bony involvement is best seen on this modality. MRI features are of a largely iso/hyperintense T1 and hyperintense T2 signal lesion which may be heterogeneous. Fluid sensitive sequences may show the triple sign: very high signal of necrosis and cystic degeneration, high signal soft tissue components, and low signal calcification or fibrotic components.

Management is largely a combination of surgery and neoadjuvant chemoradiotherapy. Small tumours in the extremities of young patients have a good prognosis. Centrally located, large tumour with haemorrhage, necrosis or poorly differentiated histology are all poor prognostic factors.

Differential diagnosis:

  x   Pleomorphic undifferentiated sarcoma
  x   Osteosarcoma
  x   Chondrosarcoma

Case 9

Dr Alistair D Calder

A 6-day-old male with a significant family history has leukopenia and hypocalcaemia. A skeletal survey is performed. What are your findings? What is the likely diagnosis?

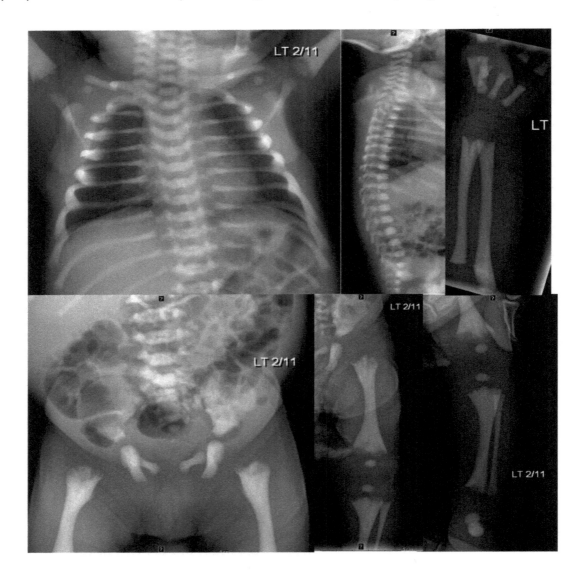

Infantile osteopetrosis

Findings: There is generalised osteosclerosis, with loss of the medullary space throughout the skeleton. There is some irregular fraying of some of the metaphyses.

Discussion: Osteopetrosis are a group of disorders resulting from osteoclast dysfunction. They are genetically heterogeneous, and range in severity from infantile forms, with a poor prognosis without treatment, intermediate forms presenting in later childhood, and adult types, which are often incidentally detected and asymptomatic. The commonest infantile type (confirmed in this case, who had an older affected sibling) is due to homozygous inactivating mutations in TCIRG1, a gene which regulates T-cell function.

Infantile osteopetrosis typically presents with pancytopenia and hepatosplenomegaly due to loss of bone marrow space. Visual loss may occur early on.

Radiological examination demonstrates generalised osteosclerosis. With time, rachitic like changes often develop in the metaphysis, reflecting impaired calcium homeostasis due to loss of osteoclast function.

TCIRG1 related osteopetrosis can be successfully treated with bone marrow transplantation if diagnosed early enough.

Radiological differential diagnoses include pyknodysostosis, which exhibits acro-osteolysis and a straight mandibular ramus, usually with less striking osteosclerosis; and physiological osteosclerosis of the newborn. Physiological osteosclerosis usually demonstrates a preservation of the marrow space and will not show haematological defects or organomegaly.

Cardiothoracic cases

Case 1

Dr Bal Sharma and Dr Aladdin Hamad

A 36-week-female infant presents with persistent right lower lobe consolidation. The patient is on CPAP.

What are the examinations and what are your findings?

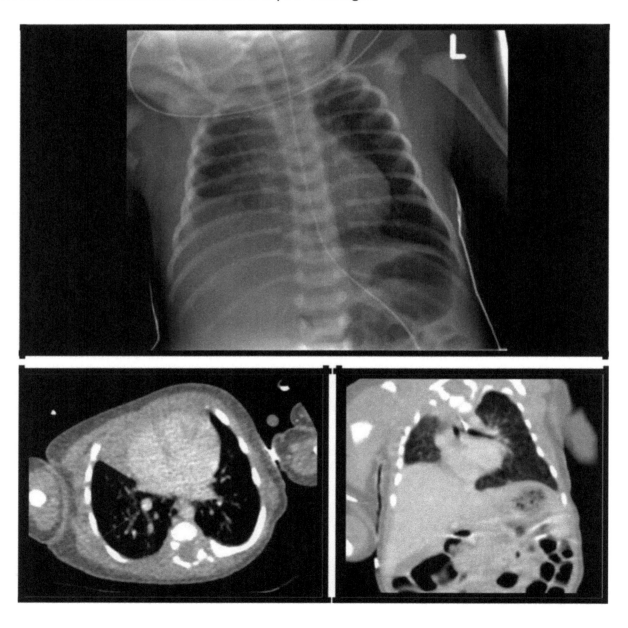

Scimitar syndrome

Findings: On the chest radiograph there is a hypoplastic right lung. This is confirmed on the CT and a large anomalous vein is seen in the right lung.

Discussion: Scimitar syndrome is characterised by a hypoplastic lung that drains via an anomalous vein into the systemic, not pulmonary, venous system. It is also known as pulmonary venolobar syndrome or hypogenetic lung syndrome and is a type of partial anomalous pulmonary venous return.

It almost exclusively occurs on the right side. The common drainage pathways of the anomalous vein are:

- x   Inferior vena cava (most common)
- x   Right atrium
- x   Portal vein

On the chest radiograph provided there is a small right lung with ipsilateral mediastinal shift. In one third of cases the anomalous draining vein is seen as a tubular structure running parallel to the right heart border in the shape of a Turkish sword ("Scimitar").

The anomalous drainage causes an acyanotic left-to-right shunt. Surgical correction is considered if there is a left-to-right shunt causing pulmonary hypertension by redirecting the pulmonary venous return into the left atrium.

There are numerous associations including:

- x   Pulmonary sequestration
- x   Congenital heart disease
- x   Ipsilateral diaphragmatic anomalies
- x   Localised bronchiectasis
- x   Vertebral anomalies

Differential diagnosis

- x   Pulmonary sequestration
- x   Right middle lobe atelectasis
- x   Unilateral absence of the pulmonary artery

Case 2

Dr Aladdin Hamad

A 33-week-old infant with intrauterine growth retardation has an increased oxygen requirement. The team are concerned the infant has a form of skeletal dysplasia.

What is the examination and what are your findings?

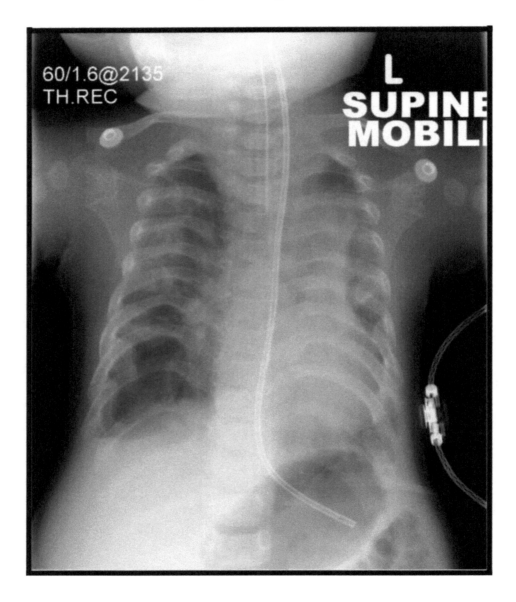

Asphyxiating thoracic dysplasia

Findings: The thoracic cavity is long and narrowed and there is an abnormal configuration of the ribs.

Discussion: Asphyxiating thoracic dysplasia or dystrophy, also known as Jeune syndrome, is a rare form of short limb skeletal dysplasia and is also sometimes classified as one of the short rib polydactyly syndromes. It is a genetically heterogeneous autosomal recessive condition with an estimated incidence of 1:70,000.

It is characterised by a long, narrow thoracic cavity; cystic renal dysplasia and skeletal anomalies. There is a significant variation in the clinical manifestation, but features include:

- x   Skeletal
    - o   Short distal limbs (acromelic dwarfism)
    - o   Narrow, elongated thorax (bell shaped)
    - o   High riding clavicles ("handlebar clavicles")
    - o   Acetabular dysplasia with flat roof and trident acetabulae
    - o   Premature closure of the capital femoral epiphysis
    - o   Short broad phalanges, coned epiphyses and polydactyly
- x   Abdominal
    - o   Cystic renal, hepatic and pancreatic disease

The prognosis is variable due to the marked variation in phenotype. Mortality is mostly due to respiratory compromise secondary to the narrow thorax, which can be complicated by pulmonary hypoplasia. In those who survive skeletal and thoracic deformities can improve during the first year of life. However, children rarely survive beyond their teenage years due to the development of renal, pancreatic and hepatic failure.

- x   Other forms of achondroplasia
- x   Thanatophoric dysplasia
- x   Achondrogenesis
- x   Cartilage-hair hypoplasia
- x   Ellis-van Creveld syndrome

Case 3

Dr Khalid Khan

A 7-year-old child presents with shortness of breath.

What are the examinations and what are your findings?

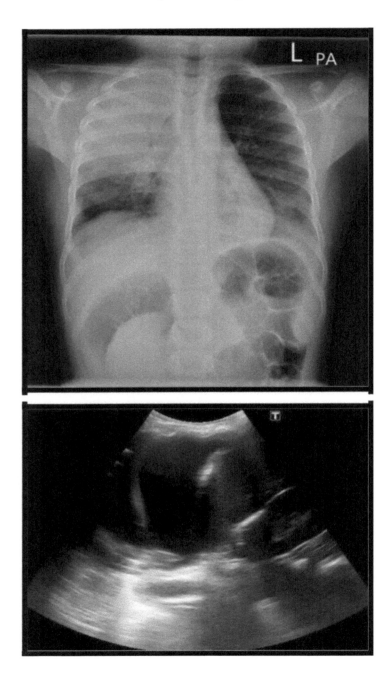

Empyema

Findings: The chest radiograph shows dense consolidation in the right upper and mid zones with an air bronchogram. There is also an even more dense rim at the upper lateral chest wall. No midline shift is seen to suggest volume loss. On ultrasound this consolidation was associated with a large loculated pleural effusion. In the setting of septations and loculations an empyema was diagnosed.

Discussion: Parapneumonic effusions can complicate pneumonia in paediatric patients. These are predominantly exudative and are termed an empyema when there is the presence of pus.

The most common causative organism in the paediatric population is *staph pneumoniae* and *staph aureus*. Group A streptococci may be seen as a complication of an infectious skin condition such as impetigo or varicella.

Differential diagnosis:

- x   Isolated pulmonary consolidation
- x   Congestive heart failure
- x   Pulmonary sequestration

Case 4

Dr Khalid Khan

A 35-week-infant was proving difficult to wean off ventilation. On auscultation the breath sounds were quiet.

What is this examination and what are your findings?

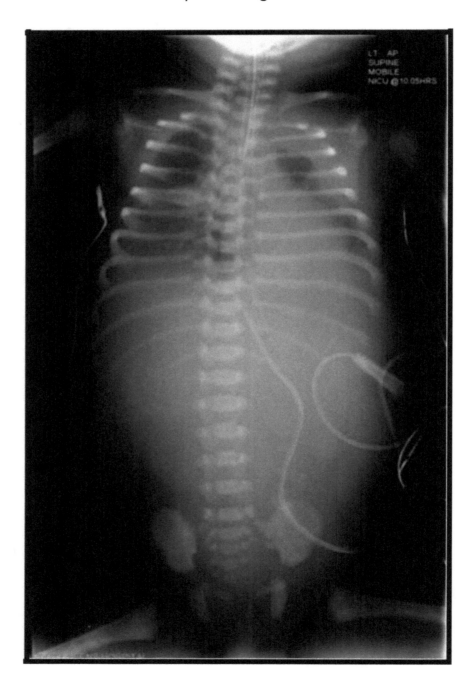

Bilateral pleural effusion

Findings: On the chest radiograph there are bilateral peripheral densities in keeping with bilateral pleural effusions.

Discussion: This case of bilateral pleural effusion in a neonate was likely due to infection. The new born was infant of a diabetic mother.

A targeted ultrasound of the right hemithorax was performed which showed a very large pleural effusion on both sides with partial collapse of the right lung posteriorly. The fluid was anechoic with no abnormal debris within it or sequestration to suggest an empyema.

Chylothorax is the most common cause of pleural effusion in the first week of life and may be acquired or congenital. Hydrops fetalis is another cause of congenital pleural effusion. Other causes in NICU are extravasation of a percutaneous central venous catheter, parapneumonic effusion and congestive cardiac failure.

Case 5

Dr Ambalika Das

A right lung abnormality was diagnosed antenatally. After birth the child had a chest radiograph and cross-sectional imaging to further characterise the lesion.

What are these examinations and what is the likely diagnosis?

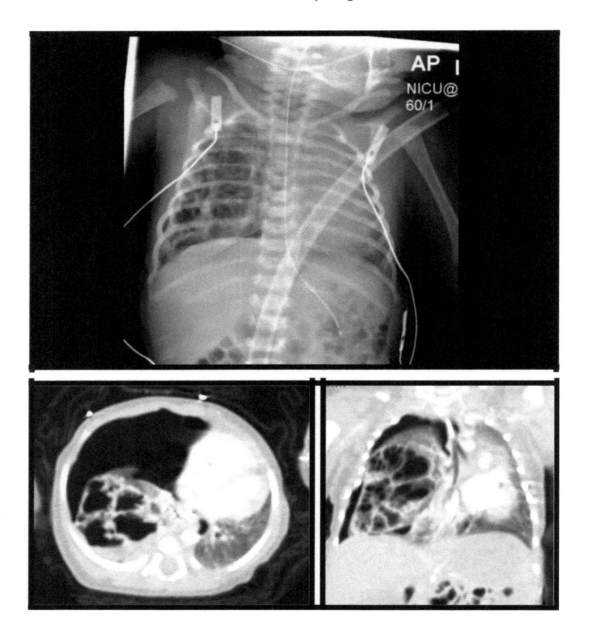

Congenital pulmonary adenomatoid malformation (CPAM)

Findings: On the chest radiograph there are bubbly lucencies occupying the right hemithorax. This is seen on the CT as a multiloculated air filled lesion in the right hemithorax with a large pneumothorax causing mediastinal shift to the left.

Discussion: CPAMs are rare adenomatous malformation of the alveoli which results in macro- or microcysts. Diagnosis is usually made on antenatal ultrasound in which it appears as a cystic or solid thoracic mass. There may be associated hydrops fetalis or polyhydramnios.

On plain radiograph it is initially a fluid-filled mass that appears solid and subsequently becomes an air-filled, multicystic lesion. In our patient there is an associated pneumothorax, which is a recognised complication.

There are five subtypes of CPAM that are organised according to cyst size. The most common is type 1 (cysts measure 2 to 10 cm). Type 2 CPAM (cysts measure < 2 cm) is more commonly associated with other anomalies such as renal agenesis, pulmonary sequestration and congenital cardiac anomalies

Treatment is usually for respiratory complications including recurrent pneumothorax and haemopneumothorax, recurrent infections and a recognised risk of malignant transformation.

Associations:

- x   Hybrid lesion: CPAM and pulmonary sequestration
- x   Renal agenesis, polyhydramnios and hydrops fetalis
- x   Lung malignancy

Differential diagnosis:

- x   Congenital pneumonia
- x   Bronchogenic cyst / pneumatocele
- x   Pulmonary sequestration
- x   Congenital diaphragmatic hernia
- x   Congenital lobar emphysema

Case 7

Dr Khalid Khan

A 2-year-old male presents with recurrent chest infections.

What are the examinations and what are your findings?

Initial study   10 days later

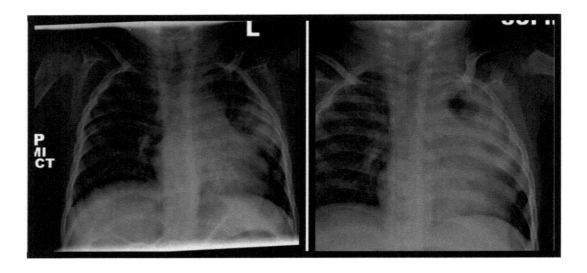

16 days later

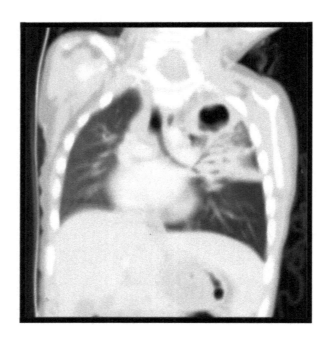

Lung abscess

Findings: On the chest radiographs there is a progressive density in the left upper zone with a central lucent area. This is also seen on the CT thorax.

Discussion: Lung abscesses are pulmonary infections that lead to destruction of the lung parenchyma and form thick-walled cavities containing pus. These may be primary or secondary (in the setting of a pre-existing lung or systemic disorder).

In primary lung abscesses the most common causative organisms are *Streptococcus pneumoniae, Staphylococcus aureus* and oral bacteria. In secondary cases the most common pathogen is *Pseudomonas aeruginosa.*

Treatment is with antibiotics with or without surgical drainage depending on whether there is a prolonged fever despite antibiotic treatment or a large abscess size.

Differential diagnosis:

- x Empyema
- x CPAM
- x Pulmonary sequestration
- x Langerhans cell histiocytosis
- x Bronchiectasis e.g. in cystic fibrosis

The following is another case of a lung abscess in a 1-year-old child with tachypnea cough and fever for more than a week.

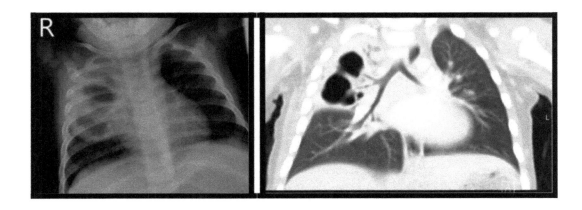

Case 8

Dr Khalid Khan

A 6-year-old girl presents with shortness of breath and chest pain. She then developed swollen, painful glands in the neck.

What are the examinations and what are your findings?

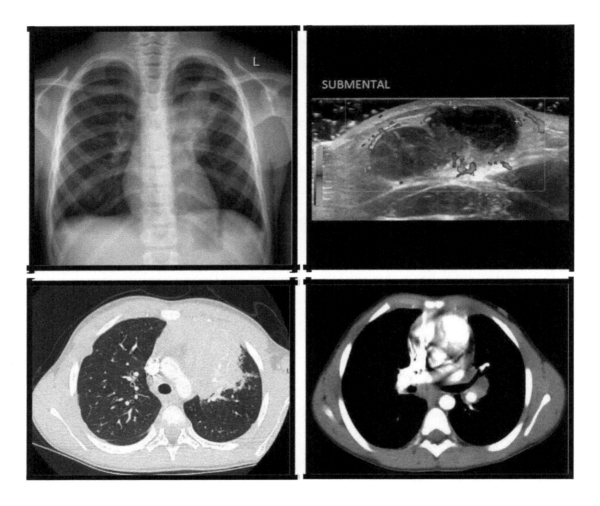

Tuberculosis

Findings: The chest radiograph shows left upper zone consolidation and the CT demonstrates additional enlarged subcarinal and left hilar nodes. On ultrasound the neck nodes are enlarged and necrotic.

Discussion: The patient had a biopsy of the submental nodes, which demonstrated florid caseating granulomas supporting a diagnosis of tuberculosis (TB).

The most common form of pulmonary TB is associated with lymphadenopathy. Progression of the lung parenchymal component can lead to progressive primary TB in which there is caseating necrosis, pneumonia and air trapping. Reactivation of TB, which has a more subacute presentation, typically occurs in older children.

Haematogenous spread may lead to miliary TB, TB meningitis and skeletal involvement. Disseminated, miliary and meningitic TB are associated with a much poorer prognosis. Other complications include pleural effusions, especially in older children, and bronchiectasis. Later complications that can develop are bronchiectasis, airway stenosis and a bronchoesophageal fistula.

Differential diagnosis:

- x Aspergillosis
- x Actinomycosis
- x Bronchiectasis
- x Pyogenic pneumonia

Case 9

Dr Khalid Khan

A 16-year-old presents with shortness of breath, a low grade, longstanding fever and weight loss.

What are the examinations and what are your findings?

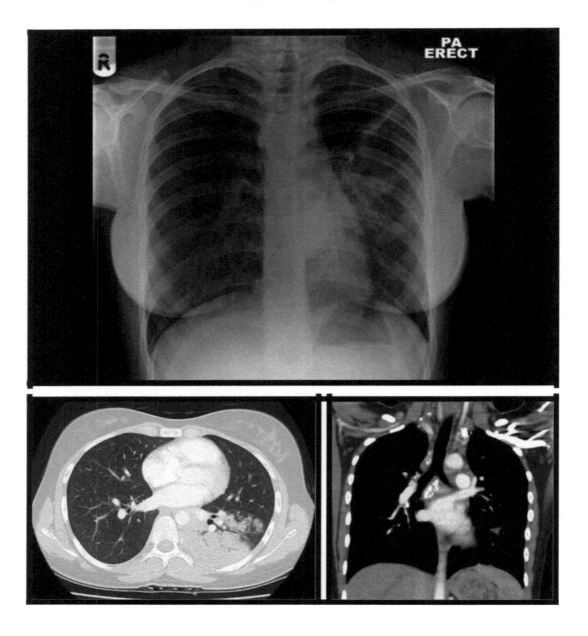

Reactivated tuberculosis

Findings: The chest radiograph shows a left retrocardiac density and left upper lobe consolidation as confirmed on the CT. Additionally, the CT demonstrates calcified mediastinal lymphadenopathy.

Discussion: The patient was diagnosed with reactivated tuberculosis. The risk of reactivation of latent TB is increased in those who are immunocompromised (e.g. AIDS/HIV, chemotherapy and systemic steroids) and have malnutrition.

Differential diagnosis of calcified mediastinal lymphadenopathy:

- x Old healed fungal infection
- x Old healed granulomatous infection
- x Metastatic osteosarcoma

Case 10

Dr Khalid Khan

The study below is from a resuscitation call for a neonate with previous cardiac surgery who presented with status epilepticus and is now non-responsive. The infant was intubated, and the team is querying an intracranial pathology.

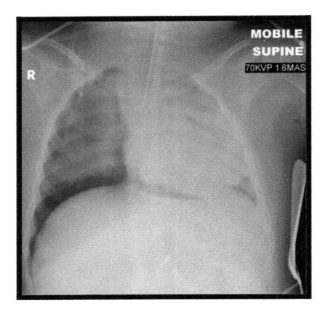

After half an hour the neonate was still unresponsive and was become more difficult to ventilate. A repeat chest x-ray was performed.

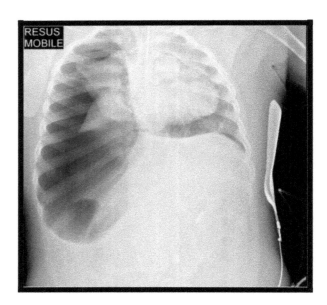

Pneumothorax and pneumopericardium

Findings: The initial chest radiograph shows gas outlining the inferior border of the heart and crossing the diaphragm in keeping with a pneumopericardium. In addition, there is a "deep sulcus sign" on the right indicative of a pneumothorax.

On the later radiograph the pneumothorax has now increased in size and is under tension as it is causing a contralateral midline shift, inversion of the right hemidiaphragm and collapse of the right lung. The pneumopericardium has also increased in size and is now outlining the entire heart but not extending beyond the level of the great vessels ("halo sign").

Discussion: Pneumopericardium may be secondary too thoracic surgery (as in this patient who has midline sternotomy wires), positive pressure ventilation, trauma, infectious pericarditis with gas-forming organisms or a fistula.

Pneumopericardium, if it increases, can cause cardiac tamponade, which decreases the cardiac return and leads to shock.

Paediatric pneumothorax may be spontaneous, for example in children with cystic fibrosis, asthma or pneumonia, or secondary to injury such has trauma, surgery or ventilation.

Tension pneumothorax is a life-threatening emergency and requires immediate decompression. If it is allowed to increase in size it can cause significant contralateral mediastinal shift, a decrease in the cardiac output and decreased venous return, which leads to shock.

Differential diagnosis of pneumopericardium:

- x Pneumomediastinum
- x Pneumoperitoneum

Differential diagnosis of pneumothorax:

- x Congenital lung malformation
- x Cystic adenomatoid malformation
- x Paediatric bronchogenic cyst

Case 11

Dr Bal Sharma

A newborn baby presents soon after birth with signs of respiratory distress.

What is this examination and what are your findings?

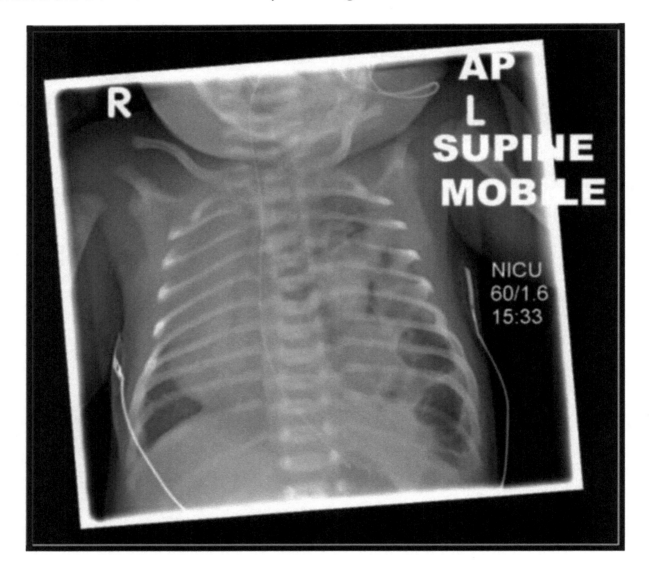

Congenital diaphragmatic hernia

Findings: The radiograph shows bubbly opacification in the thorax and mediastinal deviation to the right highlighted by the tracheal deviation.

Discussion: Congenital diaphragmatic hernias are present in 1:2000-4000 live births. They are most commonly left sided and can be classified into two subtypes:

The Bochdalek subtype is the most common. It usually occurs on the left and is in a posterolateral position. The Morgagni hernia is less common and is in an anterior position.

Associations:

- x Pulmonary hypoplasia
- x Bronchopulmonary sequestration
- x Cornelia de Lange syndrome
- x Congenital cardiac anomalies
- x Neural tube defects

If large, the hernia may cause pulmonary hypoplasia and pulmonary hypertension. Features that indicate a poor prognosis include:

- x Intra-thoracic liver
- x Small contralateral lung
- x Associated abnormalities
- x Bilateral diaphragmatic hernias

Differential diagnosis:

- x Congenital pulmonary airway malformation
- x Pulmonary sequestration

Case 12

Dr Bal Sharma and Dr Khalid Khan

A term baby presents with grunting and oxygen requirements. There was a history of meconium stained liquor at birth.

What is this examination and what are your findings?

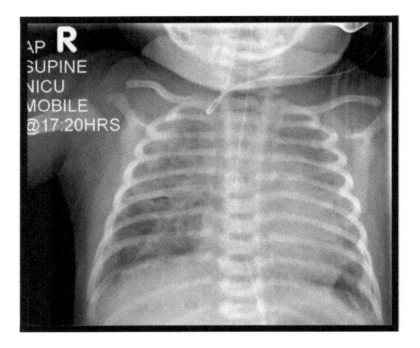

The infant continued to have difficulty in breathing and an increasing oxygen requirement. A repeat chest x-ray was performed.

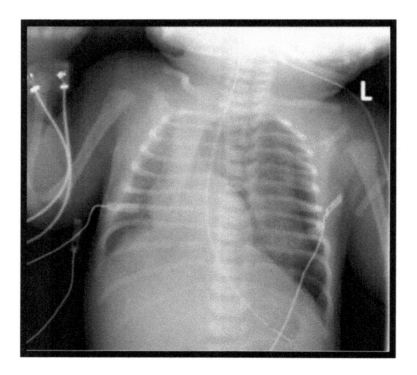

Meconium aspiration

Findings: In the initial radiograph there are rope-like perihilar densities in both lungs. On the repeat study there is a left tension pneumothorax causing mediastinal shift.

Discussion: Intrauterine passage of meconium is associated with fetal distress. During delivery a baby can aspirate amniotic fluid mixed with meconium. It is sterile but can cause pulmonary injury via several mechanisms.

1. Mechanical obstruction of the small airways can cause air trapping. On a radiograph there will be obstruction seen as collapse and atelectasis of the lungs and air trapping. The air trapping causes hyperexpanded lungs, which can lead to a pneumothorax.
2. Chemical pneumonitis
3. Pulmonary hypertension due to vasoconstriction which may lead to right-to-left shunting through the PDA
4. Increased risk of bacterial infection

Meconium aspiration syndrome (MAS) is more common in infants born at or beyond the due date. Passage of meconium in utero is usually triggered by fetal hypoxic stress. This can be triggered by placental insufficiency, maternal hypertension and preeclampsia, maternal substance abuse etc.

The clinical spectrum varies from mild to very severe. Management and outcome depend on the severity of the disease. Complications of MAS are air block syndromes (pneumothorax, pneumomediastinum, pneumopericardium), pulmonary interstitial emphysema, and persistent pulmonary hypertension of the newborn.

Differential diagnosis:

- x   Surfactant deficiency
- x   Transient tachypnea of the newborn
- x   Congenital heart disease with pulmonary hypertension
- x   Idiopathic pulmonary artery hypertension
- x   Aspiration syndromes
- x   Congenital pneumonia

Case 13

Dr Khalid Khan

A premature baby on NICU continues to have respiratory distress. The team suspects sepsis.

What is this examination and what are your findings?

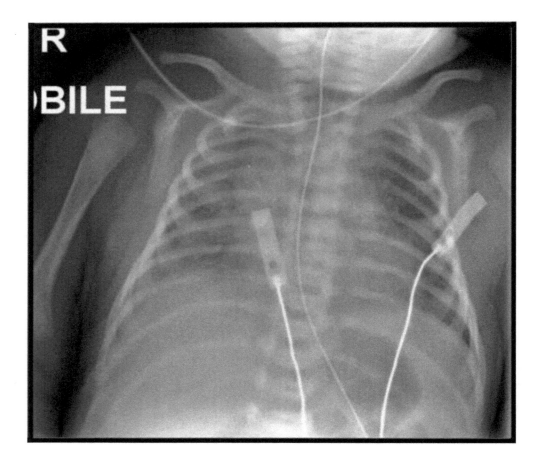

Respiratory distress syndrome

Findings: The lungs are small volume with symmetric, diffuse, ground glass opacification.

Discussion: Respiratory distress syndrome (RDS) is also known as hyaline membrane disease, lung disease of prematurity and surfactant deficiency disorder. It is due to surfactant deficiency and is more common in maternal diabetes, greater prematurity, prenatal asphyxia and multiple gestations.

A chest radiograph will show diffuse ground glass opacification, which is usually bilateral and symmetrical, and small volume lungs. There may be air bronchograms.

Treatment is with endotracheal intubation and surfactant replacement followed by invasive or noninvasive ventilation.

Acute complications are pneumothorax, pulmonary haemorrhage and treatment related (barotrauma and oxygen toxicity). More long-term complications include Bronchopulmonary dysplasia, pulmonary interstitial emphysema and recurrent pneumonia.

Below is an example of another infant with RDS who developed a pneumothorax.

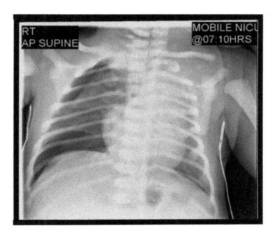

Differential diagnosis:

- x   Transient tachypnea of the newborn
- x   Congenital heart disease
- x   Pulmonary oedema
- x   Pulmonary haemorrhage

Case 14

Dr Ambalika Das

A 26-week gestation baby was delivered by emergency caesarean section due to preterm labour and foetal distress. He was intubated for 3 days then placed on biphasic CPAP. On day 9 he developed worsening respiratory acidosis and was ventilated again requiring a high pressure to ventilate the lungs effectively.

What is this examination and what are your findings?

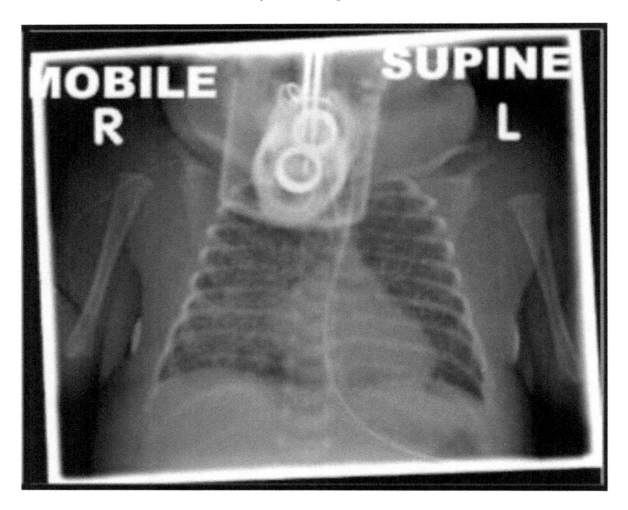

Pulmonary interstitial emphysema

Findings: There are cystic radiolucencies throughout both lungs. The lung volumes are slightly larger than to be expected for this gestation.

Discussion: Pulmonary interstitial emphysema is primarily a condition that affects the preterm surfactant deficient lung and is almost always a result of mechanical ventilation or continuous positive airway pressure. It is due to air leaking into the interstitium as a result of rupture of small airways distal to the termination of their fascial sheath.

Risk factors for development are reduced lung compliance (as is the case in surfactant deficient premature lungs), prematurity, low birth weight, meconium aspiration and pneumonia. The lung volumes are increased due to the large volume of air in the interstitium. Quite often there may be associated air-leak such as pneumothorax, pneumopericardium, pneumomediastinum or subcutaneous emphysema.

With the use of more sophisticated ventilators the incidence of PIE has decreased significantly over the years.

Case 15

Dr Ambalika Das

A 28/40 baby who was stable on low ventilator settings started deteriorating with increased respiratory support need and pinkish/red aspirate via the ETT.

Describe the x-ray findings and possible causes.

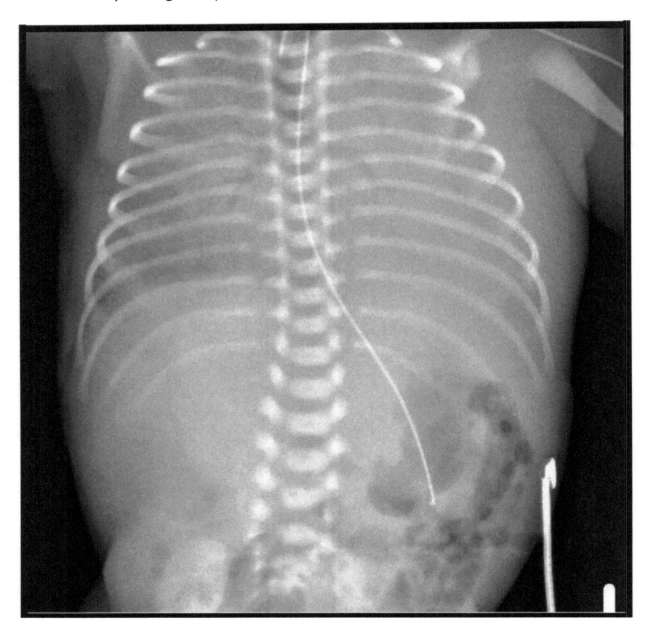

Pulmonary haemorrhage

Findings: There is bilateral diffuse dense consolidation of the lungs. Air bronchograms are seen in the perihilar region and upper zones. The aspirate findings and imaging features are in keeping with pulmonary haemorrhage.

Discussion: Pulmonary haemorrhage usually occurs on day 2 to day 4 of life in infants receiving mechanical ventilation. Exact aetiology of pulmonary haemorrhage in newborn is still unknown. It is associated with prematurity, surfactant-deficient lung disease, patent ductus arteriosus, perinatal hypoxia, hypothermia and surfactant use. It is thought that the pathophysiology involves postnatal acute left ventricular failure, which causes an increase in the filtration in the pulmonary vasculature.

Treatment includes: optimising ventilation, supportive therapy, correction of any coagulopathy, use of surfactant, management of PDA. Ventilation strategies include using higher MAP and higher PEEP on conventional mode or using higher frequency oscillation ventilation (HFOV).

Mortality can be as high as 30-40%.

Case 16

Dr Khalid Khan

A 16-year-old girl presents with a cough, fatigue and a longstanding low-grade fever.

What is this examination and what are your findings?

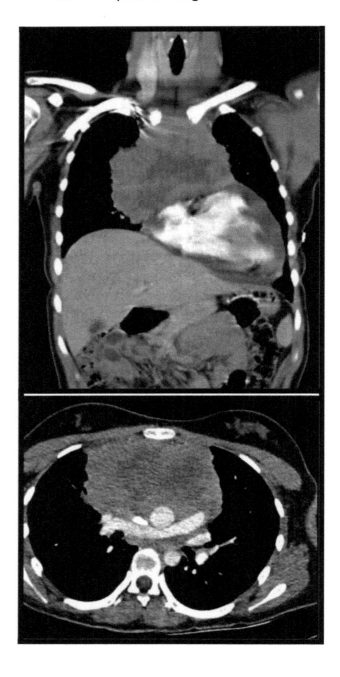

Lymphoma

Findings: The CT shows a large anterior mediastinal mass with some internal necrosis. A biopsy confirmed that this was a B-cell lymphoma

Discussion: Lymphomas are one of the most common adolescent malignancies and are broadly characterised as Hodgkin and non-Hodgkin.

Hodgkin lymphoma has a cure rate of approximately 80%. It is characterised by Reed-Sternberg cells. It is usually entirely nodal with extra-nodal disease being uncommon.

Non-Hodgkin lymphomas (NHL) are a heterogeneous group of diseases, which includes Burkitt lymphoma and lymphoblastic lymphoma. Extra-nodal disease is common. Risk factors include immunodeficiency (HIV/AIDS, post-transplant, congenital immunodeficiency syndromes) and Epstein-Barr virus.

Large mediastinal tumours can cause vascular obstruction. Other complications are mainly related to chemotherapy treatment such as growth retardation, reduced fertility, cardiac toxicity, skeletal avascular necrosis and immunosuppression.

Differential diagnosis:

- x   Tuberculosis
- x   Cat scratch disease
- x   Mononucleosis and Epstein-Barr virus infection
- x   Toxoplasmosis
- x   Histoplasmosis

The following images show another case of lymphoma with a large anterior mediastinal mass and an associated pleural effusion.

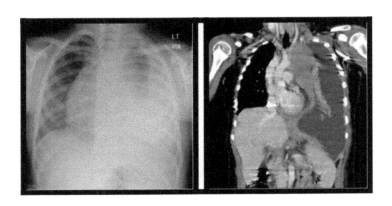

Case 17

Dr Khalid Khan

A 15-year-old boy presents with weight loss and shortness of breath.

What are the below examinations and what are your findings?

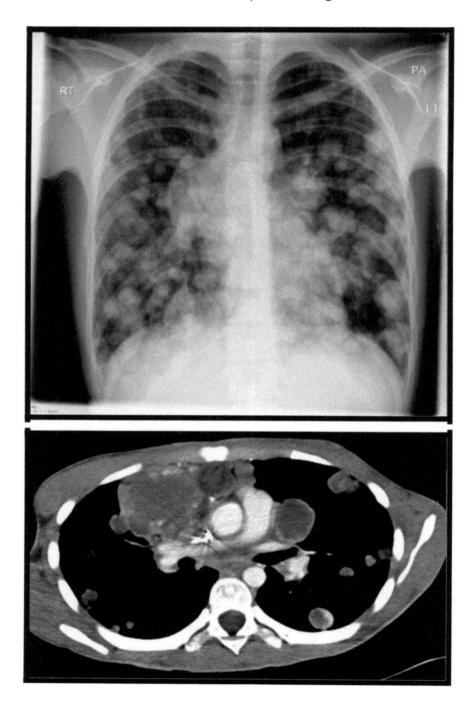

Metastatic mediastinal germ cell tumour

Findings: The chest radiograph shows a right mediastinal mass with multiple round lesions spread throughout both lungs. On the CT study the anterior mediastinal mass and the lung lesions are necrotic and show peripheral enhancement. A biopsy confirmed this to be a germ cell tumour with pulmonary metastases.

Discussion: The mediastinum is the most common extra gonadal location of germ cell tumours and, of these, 95% are in the anterior mediastinum. Germ cell tumours may be benign (mature) teratomas or malignant. Malignant lesions may be further subdivided into seminomas and non-seminomatous (also called malignant teratomas).

Mature teratomas are associated with Klinefelter syndrome. They are usually cystic and heterogeneous containing calcification, fat, fluid and soft tissue. More malignant teratomas are usually solid.

Differential diagnosis:

- x   Neurogenic tumour
- x   Thymic tumour
- x   Lymphoma
- x   Thyroid tumour
- x   Paediatric rhabdomyosarcoma

The patient was treated with chemotherapy. This was his chest radiograph two years later showing resolution of the lung nodules and mediastinal mass.

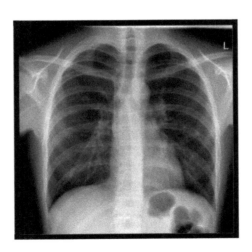

Three years after diagnosis the patient had further shortness of breath and chest pain. A chest radiograph was repeated which showed a miliary pattern of parenchymal consolidation, confirmed on the CT. The CT study also showed new lesions within the liver and kidney in keeping with metastatic disease.

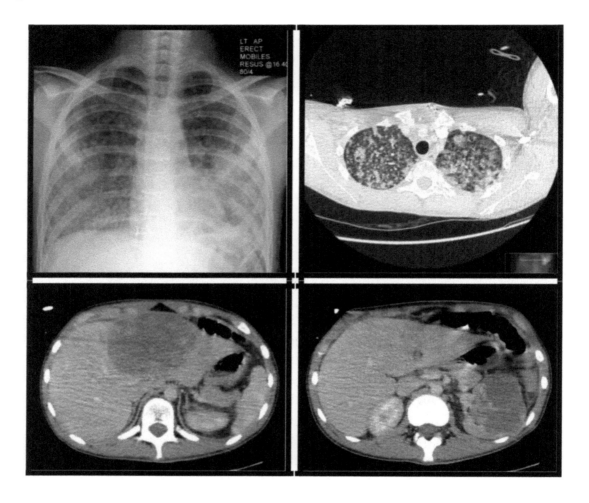

Case 18

Dr Khalid Khan

A 9-month-old child presents to A&E with difficulty in breathing and acute stridor. The child was given dexamethasone and discharged home but re-attended with continuing stridor and drooling.

What are the examinations below and what are your findings?

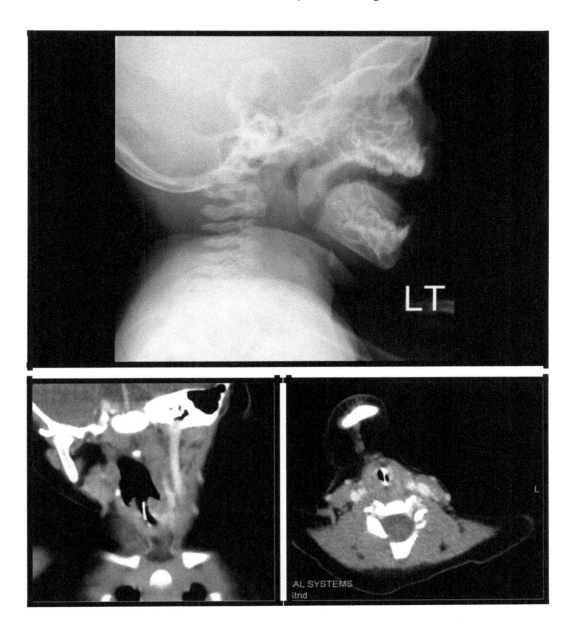

Inhaled foreign body

Findings: On the lateral neck radiograph there no opaque FB demonstrated. On CT a radiopaque linear density was seen within the hypopharynx. The mother later stated that the child started to have symptoms after being fed scrambled egg and, on surgical removal of the object, it was confirmed to be an eggshell.

Discussion: Inhaled foreign bodies are commonly seen in infants. As well as assessing the films for the presence of a foreign body it is important to assess for any associated features such as collapsed lung from objects obstructing the airway especially as many objects will not be radiopaque.

Inhaled foreign bodies are more likely to enter the right main bronchus due to it being larger and a more direct entry from the trachea than the left.

Children in whom the aspiration was not witnessed may present with persistent or recurrent cough, persistent or recurrent pneumonia and abscess, wheeze, focal bronchiectasis or haemoptysis.

Complications from swallowed foreign bodies are usually from impaction. Impaction is most likely to occur at the thoracic inlet, where the aortic arch and carina overly the oesophagus or at the lower oesophageal sphincter. Pills and button batteries may adhere to the oesophageal mucosa and pointed objects may become impaled. Once the object passes into the stomach and small bowel the risk of complications is decreased.

Differential diagnosis of inhaled foreign body:

- x Asthma
- x Bronchitis
- x Pneumonia

Gastrointestinal cases

Case 1

Dr Keir Shields and Dr Khalid Khan

A previously fit and well 13-year-old boy presented to his local walk-in-centre with a week-long history of worsening headache and an unusual rash on his legs.

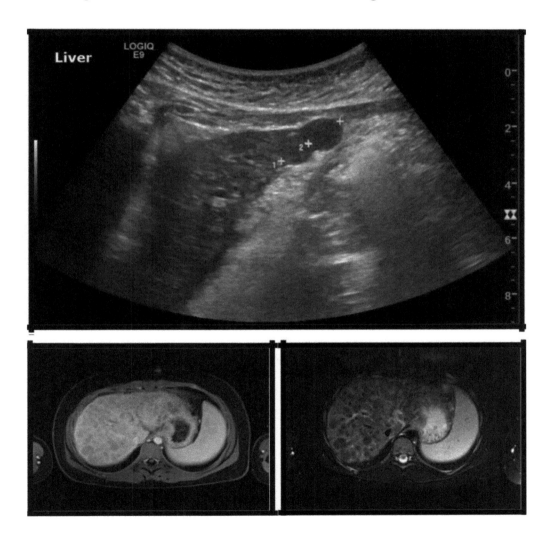

Wilson disease

Findings: On ultrasound the liver has a coarse echotexture with well-**circumscribed** nodules. The MRI confirms the irregular liver contour and more clearly displays the multiple liver nodules in all segments of the liver. These did not enhance (sequence not shown). The spleen is also enlarged.

Discussion: There are many causes of liver cirrhosis in children and adolescents. The most common in children are biliary atresia and inherited syndromes of intrahepatic cholestasis.[1] In adolescents, chronic viral hepatitis and autoimmune disease are the most common.

This was a case of Wilson disease, also called hepatolenticular degeneration, which is a rare autosomal recessive condition. It causes accumulation of copper in multiple systems including the brain, cornea, liver and, rarely, articular cartilage. Hepatic manifestations are usually after the first three years of life.

The presentation is varied and depends on the system affected and the extent of copper deposition. Symptoms include liver disease, psychiatric symptoms and movement disorders.

Treatment is with a chelating agent.

1. Santos JL, Choquette M, Bezerra JA. Cholestatic liver disease in children. Curr Gastroenterol Rep. 2010;12:30–39

Case 2

Dr Khalid Khan & Dr Benoy Starley

A 7-year-old female presents with a large abdominal mass, abdominal discomfort and weight loss.

What is the examination and what are your findings?

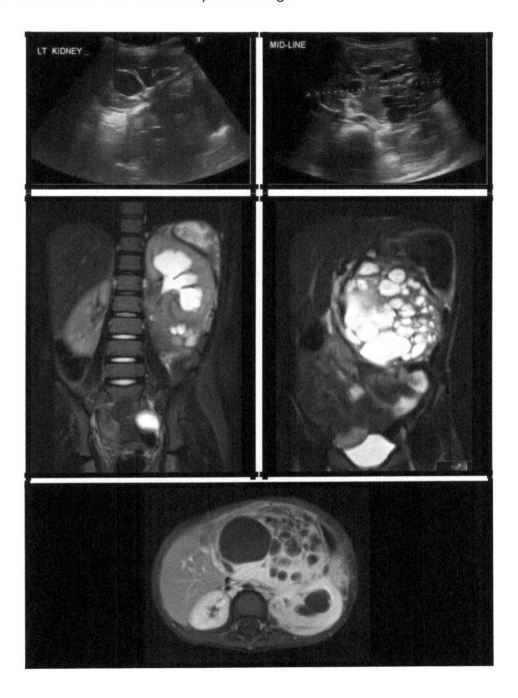

Nonrhabdomyosarcoma soft tissue sarcoma

Findings: An ultrasound of the abdomen showed a large, mixed solid and cystic, vascular mass lesion. On MRI the lesion had mass effect on adjacent organs, especially the left ureter, resulting in severe left hydronephrosis. The mass is presumed to be retroperitoneal. A sarcoma was considered, and the patient was referred to a tertiary centre. A biopsy confirmed a Nonrhabdomyosarcoma soft tissue sarcoma.

Discussion: Nonrhabdomyosarcoma soft tissue sarcomas (NRSTS) are a heterogeneous group of mesenchymal cell neoplasms. The most common subtypes are synovial cell sarcoma, fibrosarcoma and malignant peripheral nerve sheath tumour. The prognosis of NRSTSs in children is better than that in adolescents and adults.[1]

Genetic conditions such as Li-Fraumeni syndrome, Gorlin syndrome and NF1 have been associated with an increased risk of NRSTSs. Other risk factors include radiation exposure, childhood cancer and retrovirus infection in immunocompromised children.

Most NRSTSs present as painless swelling. Systemic features such as weight loss, anorexia and fever are rare.

Treatment is primarily with surgery. This may be followed up with radiation therapy or chemotherapy.

Differential diagnosis:

- x Dermatofibroma
- x Ewing sarcoma
- x Langerhans cell histiocytosis
- x Lipoma / neurofibroma
- x neuroblastoma

1. Hayes-Jordan A. Recent advances in non-rhabdomyosarcoma soft-tissue sarcomas *Semin Pediatr Surg.* 2012 Feb. 21(1): 61-7

Case 3

Dr Khalid Khan and Dr Rajesh Bagtharia

A 5-year-old male presents with persistent vomiting, dysphagia and weight loss.

What is this examination and what does it show?

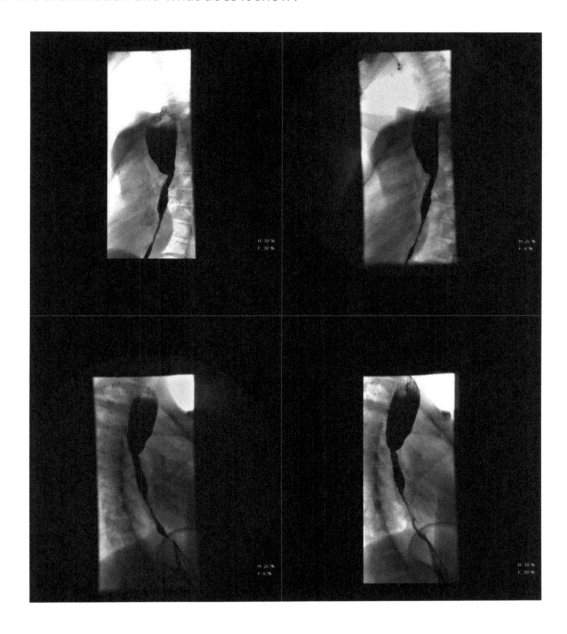

Oesophageal stricture

Findings: The barium swallow shows a persistent narrowing of the mid and lower oesophagus with poor passage of contrast through.

Discussion: Oesophageal strictures in children are most commonly due to caustic burns following the ingestion of acids or alkalis.[1] Other causes include gastro-oesophageal reflux and after surgical repair of oesophageal atresia.

Initially, after ingestion of caustic substances, there is tissue necrosis. At one-week perforation may occur if the ulceration extends through the muscle plane.

Scar retraction causing stricture formation and shortening of the involved segment usually occurs 1-3 months after the initial injury. Also, the lower gastro-oesophageal sphincter may become incompetent leading to reflux and worsening of the stricture.[2, 3]

Depending on the degree of initial injury patients may develop one or more focal strictures or more extensive stricturing as in the above case.

Management depends on the severity of the stricture and may be conservative, dilation with a stent or balloon dilatation and, in extreme cases, oesophageal replacement surgery.

1. Broor SL, Lahoti D, Bose PP, Ramesh GN, Raju GS, Kumar A. Benign esophageal strictures in children and adolescents: etiology, clinical profile, and results of endoscopic dilation. Gastrointestinal endoscopy. 1996 May; 43(5): 474-7.
2. Osman M, Russell J, Shukla D, Moghadamfalahi M, Granger DN. Responses of the murine esophageal microcirculation to acute exposure to alkali, acid, or hypochlorite. J Pediatr Surg. 2008; 43:1672–1678.
3. Mutaf O, Genç A, Herek O, Demircan M, Ozcan C, Arikan A.Gastro esophageal reflux: a determinant in the outcome of caustic esophageal burns. J Pediatr Surg. 1996; 31:1494–1495. doi: 10.1016/S0022-3468(96)901633

Case 4

Dr Khalid Khan

An 8-week-old baby presents with forceful, projectile, non-bilious vomiting.

What is the examination and what are your findings?

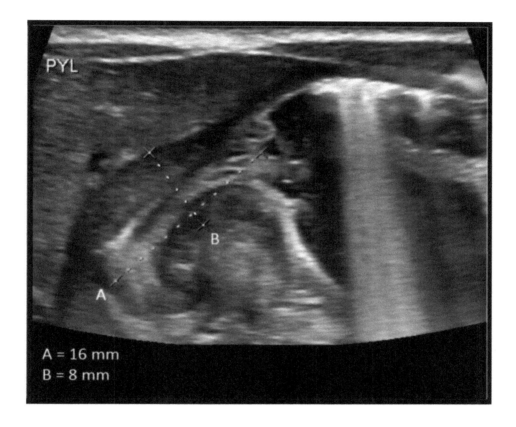

Pyloric stenosis

Findings: The ultrasound shows a thickened pylorus measuring 16 mm in length and with a pyloric wall thickness of 4 mm.

Discussion: Pyloric stenosis is a disease of unknown aetiology in which there is hypertrophy of the circular muscle of the pylorus with progressive gastric outlet obstruction. Factors associated with higher incidence are family history, male sex, and Caucasian origin. The peak age for presentation is 1 week to 3 months. Preterm infants may present later.

Infants usually present with non-bilious vomiting, which may be projectile, dehydration and failure to thrive. Hypochloremic alkalosis is the classical metabolic finding. The hypertrophic pylorus may be palpable in the right upper quadrant.

It should be noted that imaging to confirm or exclude hypertrophic pyloric stenosis is not a medical emergency. The imaging investigation of choice is an ultrasound scan. A high-frequency linear transducer (5 to 10 MHz) is used to demonstrate the enlarged pylorus in longitudinal and transverse sections.

The pylorus is located near the gall bladder, so an easy technique is to find the gallbladder and turn obliquely sagittal to the body in an attempt to visualise a pylorus longitudinally. The hypertrophic muscle is hypoechoic, and the central mucosa is hyperechoic. The pylorus is not seen to open during real-time evaluation. A normal pylorus is much harder to image then an abnormal pylorus. Over distension of the stomach pushes the pylorus posteriorly and it may be difficult to visualise. In this case a gastric tube should be inserted, and the stomach emptied.

Evidence of gastric outlet obstruction is provided by fluid filled stomach and the failure to observe any passage of fluid or air into the duodenum. A rough guide is that a pyloric length measurement of 15 to 16 mm and a muscle width approximately of 3 to 3.5 mm is indicative of pyloric stenosis.

Barium is only used if the clinical suspicion of pyloric stenosis is persistent and ultrasound is equivocal. The elongated pyloric canal can be demonstrated with shouldering of the antrum and delayed gastric emptying.

Surgery is carried out to restore normality of the pyloric canal.

Case 5

Dr Ambalika Das

A preterm neonate has developed abdominal distension, bile-stained aspirate and blood-mixed stool.

What is the examination and what are your findings?

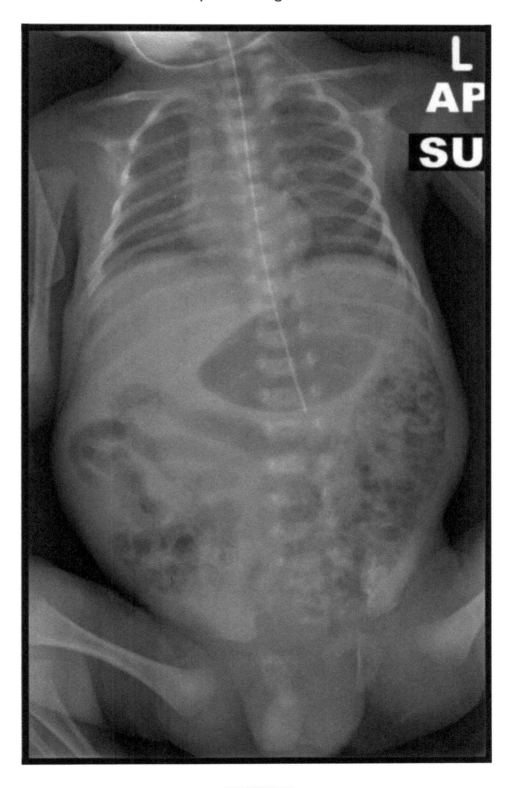

Necrotising enterocolitis (NEC)

Findings: The radiograph shows a soap-bubble appearance inside bowel cavity with linear gas shadows in the bowel wall. There is also pneumoperitoneum with the "football sign" seen in the upper abdomen.

Discussion: The radiograph shows most of the spectrum of NEC on imaging. There is pneumatosis intestinalis with gas seen in the bowel wall in the left iliac fossa. In advanced NEC this can lead to gas appearing within the portal venous system, seen as branching lucencies within the liver. There may be free intraperitoneal gas as well if there is perforation.

The aetiology of NEC is still unknown. It involves bowel inflammation, which may lead to perforation (as in this case). The risk factors include prematurity, low birth weight, intrauterine growth retardation, rapid building of feeds, formula feeds, patent ductus arteriosus etc. Premature infants are at risk of developing NEC for several weeks after birth. There may be associated sepsis and disseminated intravascular coagulation. Long-term complications include acquired short bowel syndrome secondary to surgery and stoma related complications.

Full-term or near-term infants can also develop the disease if there are predisposing factors such as perinatal asphyxia, polycythaemia, congenital anomalies etc.

Presentation may be insidious, and a high index of clinical suspicion is required. There may be gastrointestinal signs such as abdominal distension or systemic features such as respiratory failure, sepsis and circulatory collapse.

Mortality is around 50% depending on severity. The first line of treatment is conservative by stopping enteral feeds and starting broad-spectrum antibiotics. However, for cases of perforated or necrotic bowel surgery is required.

Case 6

Dr Bal Sharma and Dr Khalid Khan

A neonate has been diagnosed with possible Down's syndrome. An antenatal diagnosis of a trachea-oesophageal fistula was made. The team is worried because the infant has a distended abdomen, persistent vomiting and failure to thrive.

What is the examination and what are your findings?

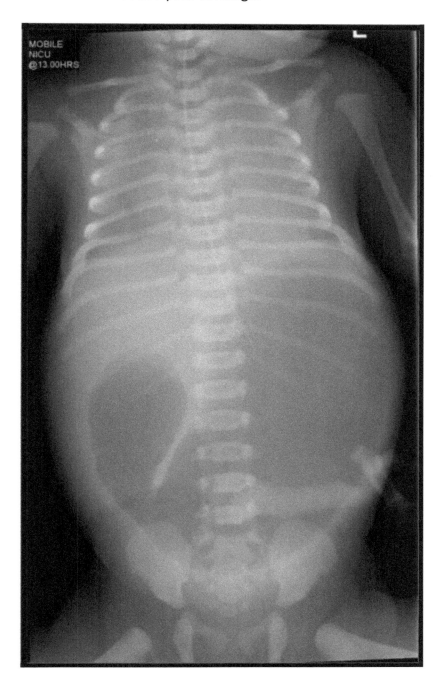

Duodenal atresia

Findings: On the radiograph a nasogastric tube is seen with the tip below the diaphragm. There is a distended gas filled structure with a "double bubble" appearance.

Discussion: Duodenal atresia occurs in 1 in 2500-5000 live births. In 25-40% of cases it is associated with trisomy 21 (Down syndrome).[1]

Many cases of duodenal atresia are diagnosed antenatally by the characteristic double-bubble sign. The first bubble corresponds to the stomach and the second to the post pyloric, prestenotic dilated duodenal loop.

Post-natally the presentation is usually as a high intestinal obstruction with bilious vomiting within hours of birth, a scaphoid abdomen, dehydration and weight loss. The neonate usually passes meconium normally.

Treatment is surgical.

Differential diagnosis:

- x Annular pancreas
- x Pyloric stenosis
- x Duodenal duplication
- x Malrotation with midgut volvulus

1. Freeman, S. B., Torfs, C. P., Romitti, P. A., Royle, M. H., Druschel, C., Hobbs, C. A., & Sherman, S. L. (2009). Congenital gastrointestinal defects in Down syndrome: a report from the Atlanta and National Down Syndrome Projects. *Clinical genetics*, *75*(2), 180-184.

Case 7

Dr Maria Lafarga

A 14-year-old female presents with an abdominal mass in the right iliac fossa after a period of fever and abdominal pain.

What is this examination and what are your findings?

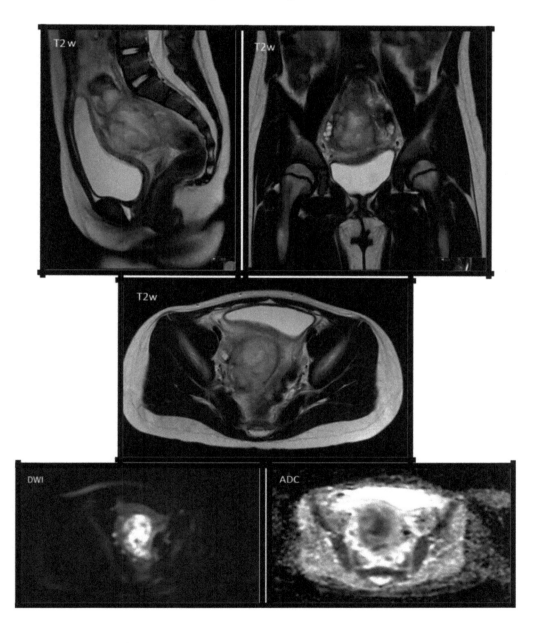

Appendicitis

Findings: The images provided show a large pelvic abnormality postero-superior to the bladder and to the right of the recto sigmoid colon, which has restricted diffusion within the abnormality.

Discussion: Appendicitis is a common cause of abdominal pain and the most common cause of a surgical abdomen in children. It occurs less frequently in infants between 2 and 5 years and is often perforated by the time the diagnosis is made.

At any age, the morbidity is secondary to complications of perforation. It is, therefore, important to make a quick and correct diagnosis of acute appendicitis.

In a minority of cases there may be findings on a plain film that point to appendicitis:

- x Appendicolith (10%)
- x Free fluid in the right lower quadrant (best seen on a prone film by separation of the colon from the properitoneal fat line)
- x Sentinel loop of bowel of localized air–fluid level in the right lower quadrant
- x Scoliosis with concavity to the right (splinting)

More recently, ultrasonography is being reliably used to diagnose a non-perforated, uncomplicated, inflamed appendix. Findings of an appendiceal width greater than 6 mm, non-compressibility of the appendix and increased vascularity are used to diagnose an acute appendicitis.

CT and MRI are more accurate and less operator dependent. The characteristic CT and MRI signs of appendicitis are a distended appendix measuring > 6 mm in diameter and an enhancing thick wall > 3 mm. In early appendicitis, the inflammatory changes may be limited to the appendiceal tip.

Findings suggesting appendiceal perforation include phlegmon, abscess, extraluminal air, an extraluminal appendicolith, and a defect in the enhancing appendiceal wall.

Phlegmons and small abscesses usually respond to antibiotic therapy alone without surgery. Large abscesses are usually managed with percutaneous drainage.

Case 8

Roger Mitcalfe and Dr Khalid Khan

A 10-month-old female presents with a three-day history of feeling generally unwell with intermittent episodes of crying, bringing up her knees and vomiting.

What are these examinations and what are your findings?

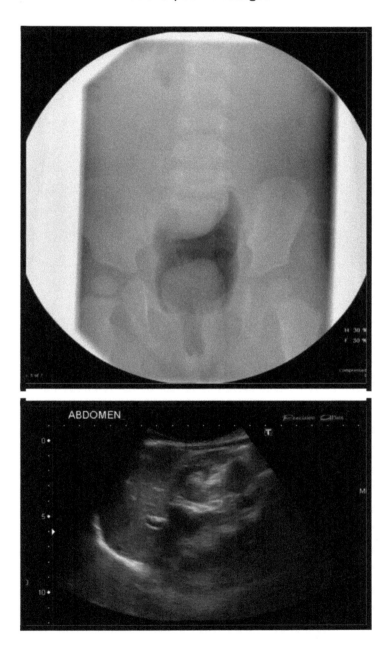

Intussusception

Findings: On the radiograph there is a dilated loop of bowel with a rounded mass protruding into the lumen. On ultrasound a "target mass" is seen with a rim of medium echogenicity and internal high echogenicity.

Discussion: Intussusception occurs when a loop of bowel invaginates into the adjacent lumen causing intestinal obstruction. Early recognition is important, as it is fatal within 2-5 days if left untreated due to bowel wall ischemia and perforation. The classic location is ileocolic. There may be a lead point that is the cause of the intussusception such as Meckel's diverticulum and lymph nodes.

Patients may present with intermittent abdominal pain, vomiting and the passage of blood and mucus, typically described as "redcurrant jelly".

Radiography will only be positive in 60% of cases. Ultrasound will show a target sign with the hypoechoic bowel wall containing another hypoechoic bowel wall in the centre and the hyperechoic omental fat in between the two. Definitive diagnosis and management is with gas insufflation under fluoroscopy guidance. If unsuccessful the patient will need surgical reduction.

Case 9

Dr Khalid Khan

An 11-year-old female presents with a two-week history of pale stools and three weeks of jaundice.

What are the investigations and what are your findings?

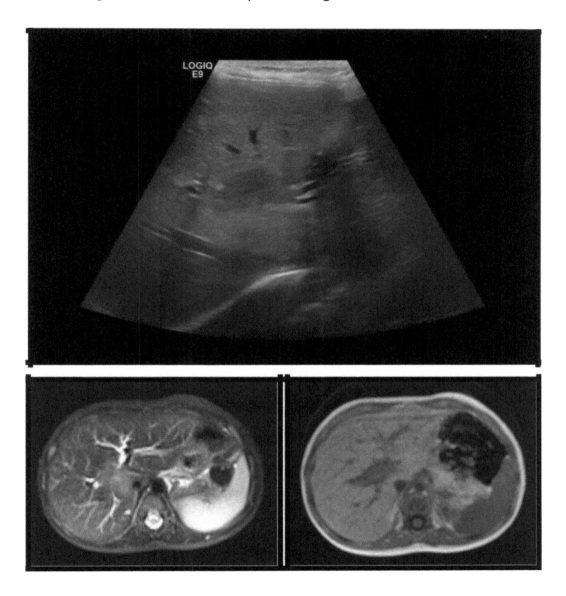

Hepatoblastoma

Findings: On ultrasound there is a hypoechoic mass in the right lobe of the liver at the confluence of the left and right portal veins. On MRI the lesion is seen as high on T2 and low on T1. There is also biliary dilation in both lobes of the liver.

Discussion: Hepatoblastoma is a malignant embryonic tumour of childhood. It can be present at birth and can present in older children up to the age of 4 years old.

Clinically there is hepatomegaly, a painless abdominal mass, and jaundice. Sometimes this is associated with nausea and vomiting, pyrexia, and anaemia.

Serum alpha-fetoprotein is usually elevated. Imaging is required to confirm the diagnosis and define the anatomical extent of the disease for preoperative planning and chemotherapy response.

On ultrasound the lesion is seen as a hypoechoic, ill-defined mass within the liver, which may have a spoke wheel appearance due to the fibrous septa that radiate from the central hub. There may be calcification causing acoustic shadowing. On CT the mass is poorly enhancing, well defined and heterogeneous with areas of calcification, haemorrhage and cystic change. Metastases occur in the lungs, para-aortic nodes and brain.

On MRI the lesion is typically high on T2 with low T2 signal fibrous bands.

Differential diagnosis:

- x Haemangioendothelioma
- x Mesenchymal hamartoma
- x Hepatocellular carcinoma
- x Neuroblastoma metastasis

Case 10

Dr Khalid Khan

A 10-year-old male presents with two months of intermittent abdominal pain.

The blood tests show deranged LFTs.

What is this examination and what are your findings?

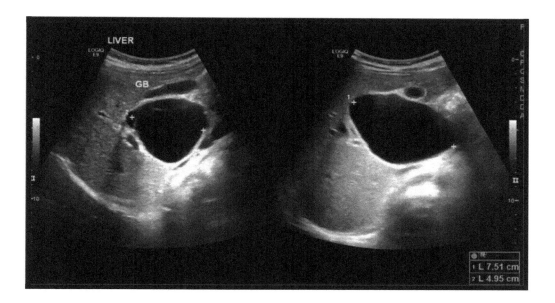

Choledochal cyst

Findings: There is a cystic structure seen inferior to the gallbladder. The remainder of the liver shows no focal lesions.

Discussion: Choledochal cysts are cystic dilatation of the common bile duct and/or the intrahepatic biliary ducts. Todani described five subtypes as follows:

- x   Type I – dilatation of the common bile duct is the most common
- x   Type II – diverticulum of a normal calibre CBD
- x   Type III – choledochocele of the intramural CBD
- x   Type IV – dilatation of the CBD and intrahepatic bile ducts
- x   Type V – dilatation of the intrahepatic bile ducts with a normal calibre CBD

The prevalence of choledochal cysts varies across populations but they are more common in Japan and Asia.

Two-thirds of cases are diagnosed before the age of ten and there are two distinct groups depending on the age at presentation. The first is the infantile group in which children younger than 1-year present with or without obvious hepatomegaly with obstructive jaundice. The second is children over 1 year who more commonly have one or more of the classic triad of pain, jaundice and a palpable mass. The jaundice is usually intermittent.

Treatment is with total excision of the cyst.

Urogenital cases

Case 1

Dr Khalid Khan

A 5-year-old male presents with microscopic haematuria.

What is this examination and what are your findings?

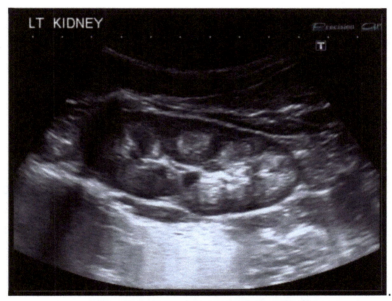

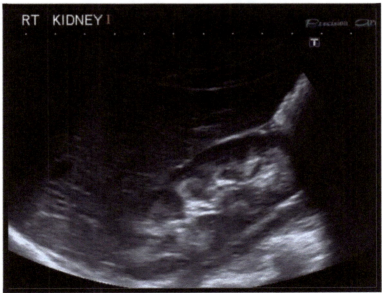

Medullary nephrocalcinosis

Findings: The ultrasound shows a large difference in the echogenicity of the medulla and cortex due to an increased echogenicity of the medullary region of the kidneys.

Discussion: Nephrocalcinosis is defined as deposition of calcium compounds within the renal parenchyma. 90% of nephrocalcinosis occurs in the medullary pyramids, which rarely cause posterior acoustic shadowing. Less often, nephrocalcinosis occurs in the renal cortex and is seen as linear cortical calcifications. Normally in the paediatric patient the medullary pyramids are hypoechoic compared to the renal cortex. In patients with nephrocalcinosis the renal pyramids are hyperechoic with reversal of the normal cortical medullary renal echogenicity relationship.

There are multiple causes of nephrocalcinosis and the majority associated with hypercalcemia. The most common causes include long-term furosemide therapy in neonates. The other causes of medullary calcinosis are renal tubular acidosis, hyperthyroidism, Williams syndrome, prolonged immobilisation, steroid therapy and hypophosphataemia

An ultrasound of a normal kidney at this age (left) is shown to highlight the abnormal echogenicity in medullary nephrocalcinosis (right).

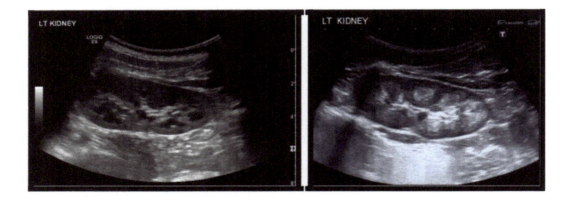

Case 2

Dr Khalid Khan

An 11-month-old boy presents with recurrent urinary tract infections.

What is this examination and what are your findings?

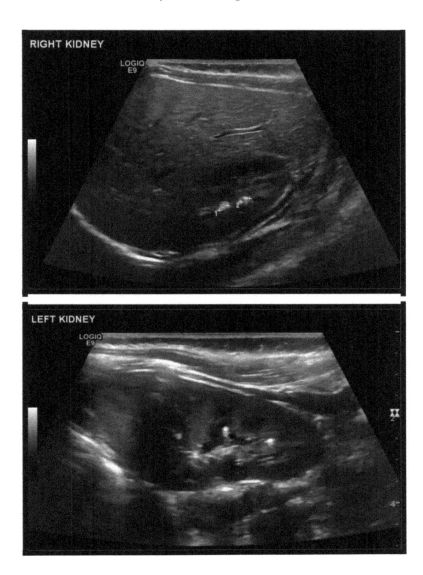

Bilateral renal calculi

Findings: There are multiple bilateral echogenic foci in the kidneys. These represent renal calculi.

Discussion: The incidence of renal calculi in children of this age group is rare in the developed world and in children of African descent.

Paediatric renal calculi are often associated with a metabolic abnormality, most commonly hypercalciuria. Functional or mechanical obstruction within the genitourinary tracts predisposes children to calculi formation due to stasis and infection. Genitourinary abnormalities such as hydronephrosis, duplex ureter, posterior urethral valves and bladder extrophy are found in a third of cases. Premature infants are also at higher risk of developing renal calculi usually due to a combination of immature renal function and medication.

The most common presenting feature is abdominal pain and gross haematuria. Recurrent urinary tract infections are also common, and patients should have the urine tested for infection. The typical colicky flank pain that adults normally present with this is rare in paediatric nephrolithiasis.

Ultrasound is the preferred initial imaging modality. If the stones are not seen on ultrasound but there remains clinical concern, then proceeding to a CT is reasonable.

Case 3

Dr Khalid Khan

A 5-month-old male baby is admitted for recurrent urinary tract infection.

What are these examinations and what do they demonstrate?

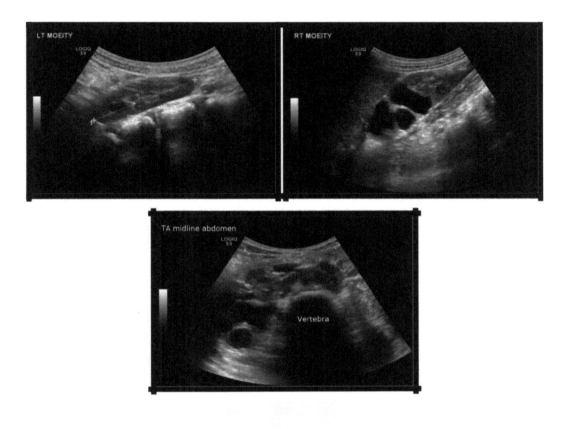

POSTERIOR

Horseshoe kidney

Findings: The ultrasound shows a normal appearance of the left kidney. In the right kidney there is dilation of the collecting system of the upper moiety and some renal tissue seen crossing the midline. The nuclear imaging confirms renal tissue crossing the midline with a non-functioning right upper moiety. The crossing midline renal tissue is characteristic of a horseshoe kidney.

Discussion: This malformation represents fusion of the kidneys resulting in lack of normal migration. It is quite frequent and is found in 1 in 500-1000 autopsies. The kidneys are more medially orientated with fused lower poles anterior to the aorta and inferior vena cava. Often several renal arteries supply the kidneys from the aorta and a range of abnormalities is seen from a thin fibrous bridge to a single pelvic renal complex with symmetrical or asymmetrical fusion.

The more distorted form generally presents quicker as they are prone to ureteropelvic obstruction, vesicoureteral reflux, stones and ureteral duplication. They frequently have an extra renal pelvis, which should not be confused with hydronephrosis. Their anterior position makes them more prone to traumatic injury.

There is an association with trisomy 18, imperforate anus, Turners syndrome and infants of diabetic mothers. When they are found clinically in the absence of these abnormalities, they have an increased incidence of congenital cardiac anomalies.

Case 4

Dr Khalid Khan

An antenatal ultrasound showed a dysplastic right kidney. The neonate is re-imaged following birth.

What are these examinations and what do they show?

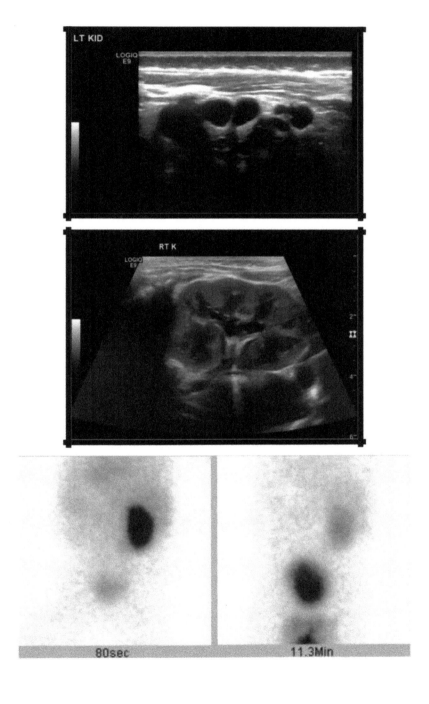

Multicystic dysplastic kidney (MCDK)

Findings: On the ultrasound left kidney there are numerous non-communicating hypoechoic cysts of varying sizes with echogenic thinned renal parenchyma. No recognisable cortical medullary differentiation is evident. The nuclear image (DMSA) shows no functioning renal tissue on the left.

Discussion: Multicystic dysplastic kidney is the second most common cause of an abdominal mass in the neonate. This non-hereditary condition is usually discovered on the prenatal ultrasound. The kidney is non-functioning and is replaced by multiple cysts of varying sizes. There is no cortical medullary differentiation and the renal contour may be preserved. This condition usually involves the entire kidney but occasionally it may be confined to one segment of the kidney. The multicystic dysplastic kidney may sometimes appear as a solitary cystic mass. Calcification can sometimes be seen in the cyst wall. 40% of patients have contralateral abnormality.

Differential diagnosis:

- x   Hydronephrosis
- x   The Wilms tumour
- x   Tuberous sclerosis
- x   End-stage renal disease
- x   Congenital mesoblastic nephroma

Management is non-operative as the cysts tend to involve with time as shown in the below ultrasound which was performed one year later.

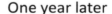

One year later

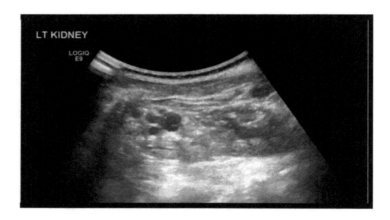

Case 5

Dr Khalid Khan

Antenatal scanning shows a multicystic left kidney. The neonate is imaged after birth.

What are these examinations and what are your findings?

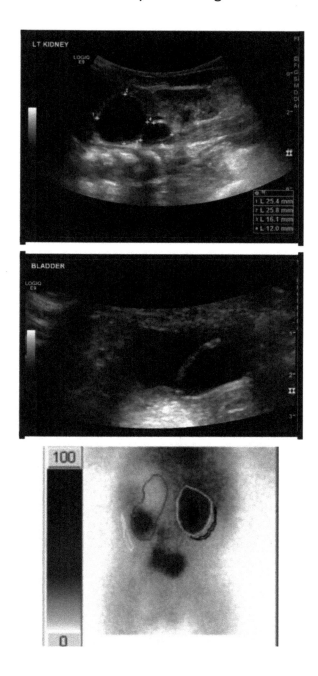

Duplex collecting system

Findings: On the ultrasound the left kidney has hydronephrosis of the upper moiety with a normal appearance of the lower moiety. A ureterocele is seen to the left of the bladder. On nuclear imaging no, functioning renal tissue is demonstrated in the upper moiety of the right kidney.

Discussion: A duplex collecting system encompasses a range of parenchymal, pelvic and ureteric duplication. It is a common congenital abnormality of the renal tract. There is incomplete fusion of the upper and lower moieties with variable duplication of the collecting system.

Where there is complete duplication of the ureters the upper pole more commonly obstructs due to a ureterocele and the lower pole moiety more commonly becomes hydronephrotic due to reflux via an ectopic ureter.

The following is another case of a duplex left kidney in which the separate renal pelvises can be clearly seen.

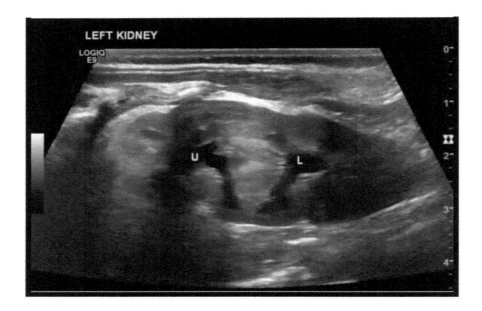

Case 6

Dr Khalid Khan

A 7-year-old girl has been complaining of pain in the right lower abdomen for several weeks.

What are the examinations and what are your findings?

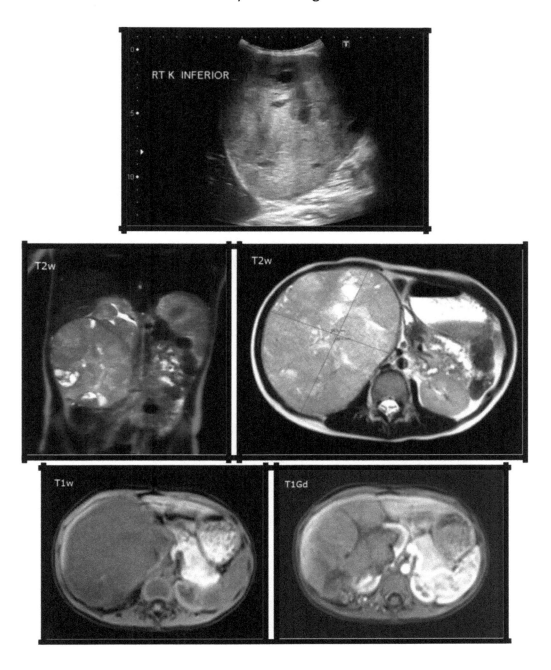

Wilm's tumour

Findings: On ultrasound there is a large solid mass, which lies inferior to the liver. On MRI a large abdominal soft tissue mass is confirmed which enhances heterogeneously. The mass invades the upper pole of the right kidney. The findings are consistent with a tumour, which was later confirmed to be a Wilm's tumour.

Discussion: Wilm's tumour, also known as nephroblastoma is a malignant renal tumour that occurs in a paediatric population. This is the most common cause of a paediatric renal mass with a peak incidence at 3 to 4 years of age. If this is part of a syndrome (e.g. Beckwith-Wiedemann syndrome) it can present even earlier.

Haemorrhage and necrosis are common. They usually displace, rather than invade, adjacent structures. Metastasis may be seen in the lung, liver and local lymph nodes and the tumour may invade into the renal vein, IVC and right atrium in advanced disease.

Treatment is mainly surgical with chemotherapy. Cure is possible in approximately 90% of cases.

Differential diagnosis:

- x   Neuroblastoma
- x   Multilocular cystic renal tumour
- x   Clear cell sarcoma
- x   Renal rhomboid tumour
- x   Angiomyolipoma

Case 7

Dr Khalid Khan

An x-ray was performed on a neonate to look at the long line placement.

What is this examination and what are your findings?

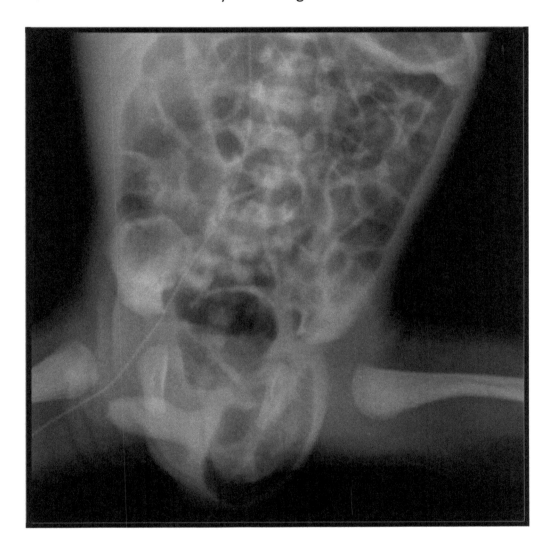

Inguinal hernia

Findings: On the plain film bowel and air can be seen in the left scrotum in keeping with a left inguinal hernia.

Discussion: Inguinal hernias are common in the paediatric population. As the processus vaginalis, the outpouching of the peritoneum attached to the testes descends into the scrotum, may not obliterate fully and this will result in a direct tract via the inguinal canal into the scrotum. In females the ovaries do not leave the pelvic cavity. Instead, there may be a tract into the labium major known as the canal of Nuck. Premature infants are more at risk of inguinal hernias.

Contents of the abdominal cavity including fluid and bowel can herniate through the 'patent canal'. Bowel, which herniates through, may become incarcerated or strangulated and lead to obstruction and necrosis. In paediatric patients with bowel obstruction it is important to include the pelvis on a radiograph to assess for an incarcerated inguinal hernia.

Inguinal hernias do not heal spontaneously and must be surgically repaired due to the risk of bowel incarceration.

The ultrasounds below show a loop of bowel within the inguinal canal(left) as well as fluid within the canal in keeping with an encysted hydrocele(right).

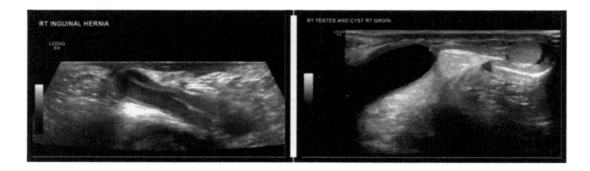

Case 9

Dr Khalid Khan

A 7-year-old boy presents with abdominal pain and a right scrotal swelling.

What is this examination and what are your findings?

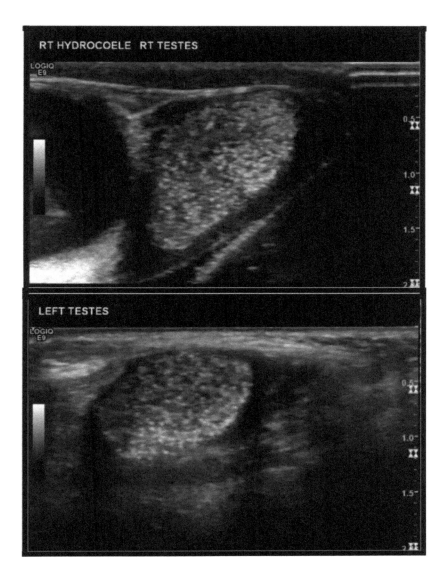

Microlithiasis

Findings: The ultrasound shows multiple bilateral punctate hyperechoic foci within the testes. This is in keeping with testicular microlithiasis.

Discussion: There are a few known associations of microlithiasis including testicular germ cell tumour, Klinefelter syndrome, cryptorchidism, Down syndrome and testicular infarct. Although microlithiasis is present in 50% of men with germ cell tumours, it is also a very common finding in the asymptomatic population.

The European Society of Urogenital Radiology advises annual follow-up ultrasound up to age 55 only if the following risk factors are present:

- x Personal / family history of germ cell tumour
- x Maldescent
- x Orchidopexy
- x Testicular atrophy

Case 10

Dr Khalid Khan

A 14-year-old-girl presents with abdominal pain and distension. On palpation there is a large abdominal pelvic mass.

What is this examination and what are your findings?

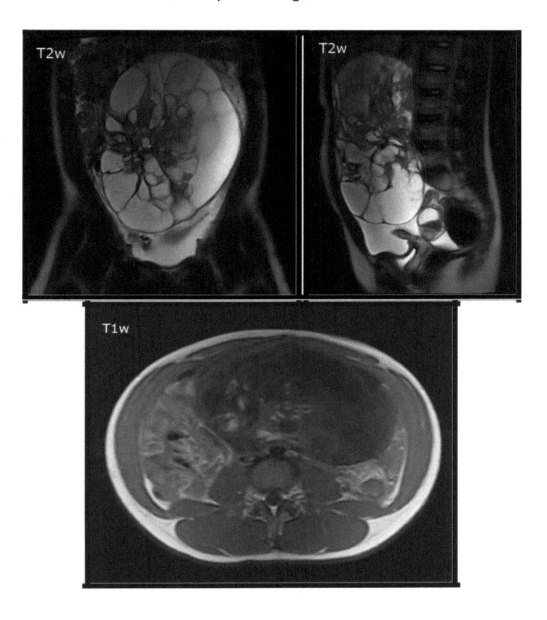

Germm cell tumour

Findings: The MRI shows a large multiloculated cystic lesion, which appears to be extending from the right adnexa. There is a high T1 signal in keeping with blood products. Ascites is also noted. The findings are in keeping with an ovarian cystic mass.

Discussion: Ovarian neoplasms in the paediatric population are uncommon. These may be benign or malignant. A solid component is the most significant indicator of malignancy.

Germ cell tumours, such benign mature teratomas (dermoids) are the most common cause of paediatric ovarian masses. The presence of fat or calcification is diagnostic. Some teratomas may contain immature components that can spread, especially to the peritoneum.

Other germ cell tumours include dysgerminoma, yolk sac tumour and choriocarcinoma.

Ovarian masses predispose to ovarian torsion, a surgical emergency.

Because of this, masses are usually treated with surgery.

Index

CPSIA information can be obtained
at www.ICGtesting.com
Printed in the USA
BVHW021212290321
603633BV00011B/1929

9 781786 233080